A History of Medicine

Selected Readings

Edited by Lester S. King

Penguin Books

Penguin Books Ltd, Harmondsworth,
Middlesex, England
Penguin Books Inc., 7110 Ambassador Road,
Baltimore, Md 21207, USA
Penguin Books Australia Ltd,
Ringwood, Victoria, Australia

First published 1971
This selection copyright © Lester S. King, 1971
Introduction and notes copyright © Lester S. King, 1971

Made and printed in Great Britain by
Richard Clay (The Chaucer Press) Ltd,
Bungay, Suffolk
Set in Monotype Times

Penguin Education

A History of Medicine

Edited by Lester S. King

History of Science Readings

Contents

Introduction

In the past thirty years medicine has made stupendous scientific advances – with new drugs and operative procedures, new diagnostic techniques, sophisticated engineering newly applied to medical problems, new concepts of delivering health care. At the same time, statistics indicate that perhaps 90 per cent of all the scientists that ever lived are alive today. It is not surprising, therefore, that medicine is making such progress. But current achievements may blind us to the merits of the past. Indeed, some dissenters even feel that the vaunted improvements in medicine are partly illusory, and that the past, with its relative paucity of scientists, is far more important than usually recognized.

We see the lack of historical feeling when we try to elicit some appreciation of the medical past. Today's medical students, for example, intent on learning the latest teachings, for the most part regard any medical writing more than twenty years old as ancient history. Furthermore, when they do happen to look backward they regard the past with distorted vision, with a viewpoint severely limited by present-day concepts. This process is sometimes called 'presentism', i.e. applying present-day standards and values to eras when quite different modes of thought pertained, quite different cultural patterns and philosophic outlook. Presentism, ignoring the cultural environment of times past, fails to relate the practices, discoveries and evaluations of a given era to its whole cultural *milieu*. Instead there is only a short-range view, like a photograph taken with a very short-focus lens. What is close to the camera is disproportionately large and what is a little way removed seems extraordinarily small.

We call this a distortion, yet the camera does not lie. It faithfully imprints on the film the scene as recorded through a particular lens. The difficulty is that the lens is not adapted to its goal. If we want to see things in a more realistic relationship, we must get optical equipment that will provide a proper perspective. So it is with the attitudes to history. We must try to replace presentism with a better 'lens'.

To appreciate past events, we should enter into the culture of the past. Psychiatrists, for example, study cultural patterns. By so doing, they find that behaviour which might appear abnormal by one set of standards can find a rational explanation when viewed relative to its own cultural environment. This is indeed a commonplace in psychiatric training. I wish it could become equally commonplace in studying medical history.

At first glance the medical doctrines of our ancestors may sound bizarre. The outlandish remedies – the purgings, bleedings and vomits – and the gullibility may appear grotesque. Quite often the reaction to all this is ridicule. A second attitude, however, avoiding ridicule, evaluates the remedies of our ancestors and finds merit therein, *but only to the degree that these findings anticipate present-day practices*. Both of these reactions, I believe, are wrong.

If we want to reconstruct the intellectual framework of times gone by, we must accept one basic proposition: that physicians then were just as intelligent as we are today, just as earnest and devoted and conscientious. To think of ourselves as clear thinking and capable, and our ancestors as benighted, is arrogance. If we accept the proposition that they were not stupid, then their concepts and pronouncements, however absurd they may seem, must have had a sound explanation in the intellectual and cultural *milieu* of their times.

Any particular concepts, taken from the past, may be false by our present-day standards. But since this concept was elaborated by persons as intelligent as we, we should inquire about the factors which induced them to make such statements. What do we need to know in order to perceive that a statement, seemingly absurd, is actually thoroughly reasonable? What was the operative background out of which this concept arose?

Medical history describes the doctrines of physicians, their observations and interpretations, activities and procedures and, equally important, the material and intellectual environment out of which these doctrines and activities arose. Medical history must describe the factors that have determined the attitudes and behaviour of physicians, their discoveries, concepts and activities. A history of medicine which restricts itself to narrative of great medical discoveries has limited interest, and deservedly so. The history of medicine, however, becomes fascinating when it relates to the cultural and intellectual patterns that have acted upon physicians and patients alike. These patterns involve such topics as basic philosophy; political, social and economic factors; literature and art in their broad senses; natural science and the investigations into the workings of nature. All are relevant to medicine.

Any single text can take up only a small fragment of the total. Since a truly comprehensive history is obviously too vast to encompass, I want to take up one limited area. In this volume I wish to indicate the development of *critical thinking* among physicians, from early times to the present. How have physicians studied nature? How have they investigated disease? How have they reached conclusions? Physicians, trained to observe, have always reflected on their observations and directed their reflections and inferences to the care of the patient or else to goals more general and theoretical, e.g. understanding the nature of health and disease. In this continuing process what have physicians accepted as 'fact'? What evidence did they consider valid? What did they ignore? What presuppositions did they accept as valid? How justifiable were their inferences? These aspects of medicine, concerned with attitudes and methods, with evidence and its evaluation, are intangibles quite distinct from the actual substantive achievements we ordinarily think of as 'medical history'.

During twenty-five centuries the attitudes of physicians have repeatedly changed, often in a cyclical or recurrent form. Various epithets, such as 'rationalism' or 'empiricism', 'mechanism' and 'vitalism', crop up again and again, although with new meanings and implications. Different metaphysical backgrounds have succeeded one another and have influenced the thought modes of physicians. 'Medical thought' involves not so much what physicians have actually discovered, but the *way that they approach their problems*, and the attitudes they manifest. Occasionally, physicians have quite deliberately analysed their own methods but for the most part they have not been self-conscious about their methodology. We discover their modes of thought and attitudes chiefly by indirection, by writings which, intended to serve other purposes, give clues to basic attitudes and approaches. And we appreciate these basic attitudes when we look at them against a background of the dominant philosophies and cultural patterns.

There are many ways of analysing the past. The historian, for example, may expound and interpret the primary sources and try to draw relationships and trace interconnections. Or he may offer an anthology of the primary sources to the reader who is thus invited to draw his own relationships and make his own interpretations. The historian, by his selection and comments, directs attention to those aspects which he considers important and thus, in a sense, is imposing his own interpretation on the reader. But the reader, examining the original sources, sometimes draws conclusions quite different from the historian's intent. After all, the past is ever new; no two people regard it with the same eyes. The historian, whether offering a straight exposition or an anthology with commentary, should try to make explicit his own personal viewpoint.

In this book I have made no attempt to pick out the 'greatest' physicians in history, nor have I tried to narrate the 'great' discoveries nor emphasize 'high spots' of medical progress. Instead, I try to illustrate methods and thought-modes of representative physicians, from Hippocrates to the present. As we go from one physician to another, we see some of the changes that have taken place, but we also find a strong kinship between good physicians of all eras. A good physician is characterized at all times by a quality which I would call 'critical acumen', even though the definition of this quality might change from one era to another. The subtitle of this volume might be, 'A study of critical acumen.'

The classical heritage

Western medicine, like western civilization as a whole, had its foundation in ancient Greek culture whose concepts have permeated all subsequent civilization. Much of what today seems new can be traced back directly or indirectly to Greek beginnings, or can be found implicit in the works of Greek thinkers. In the medicine of antiquity there were wide ranges of theory and practice, from crude superstition to high sophistication. Of course, the period that we designate as antiquity embraced approximately one thousand years from, say, the sixth century BC to the fourth century AD, and during this period we would naturally expect a tremendous sweep of thought and action, in medicine as in any other activity.

Greek medicine was a remarkable blend of observation and inference, of concrete and abstract, practical and theoretical. It was intimately related to philosophy. In classical times philosophy embraced all knowledge, speculative as well as more experiential. The Greeks were intensely concerned with the ultimate elements which comprised the universe, but these ultimate elements were considered differently by different early philosophers. The development and interplay of different conceptual schemata belongs to the history of philosophy, although for our purposes we can emphasize the importance of such metaphysical concepts in determining medical theory. The schema that won most approval analysed things into the components of air, earth, water and fire, associated with which were the primary qualities of hot, cold, moist and dry.

In addition to the speculative bent which sought the ultimate components of the universe through exercise of reason, there was also a strong empirical trend, wherein physicians paid close attention to concrete experience. This is particularly evident in the writings of Hippocrates, who observed carefully and tried to remain at all times close to concrete observation rather than jump to ultimate conclusions. Hippocrates – as I indicate later, the name undoubtedly covers many different writers – also indulged in speculation, but did so on a level considerably short of the ultimate metaphysics of the universe.

Greek thought was logical. 'Reason', a word easy to use but hard to define, served as a key to unlock the secrets of the universe. 'Reason' formed an eternal dialectic with 'experience', and this opposition has persisted throughout the history of thought. Neither reason nor experience is meaningful without the other, but the two together set up tensions, where first one would predominate, then the other. In medical history, Hippocrates represents the dominance of experience, but tempered by reason and rational inference. Hippocrates, with his well-balanced attitudes, is often contrasted with the philosophers who followed reason even when it actually contradicted experience.

In less than two hundred years Greece developed the most important metaphysical systems in western thought. Two of these – the atomistic and the Platonic approaches – form the historic foundations of medicine and, like 'rationalism' and 'empiricism', make up another of the dialectic tensions that underlie the progress of medicine.

Atomism, associated with Democritus and Lucretius, held that the ultimate stuff of the universe consists of an infinity of indestructible particles which can vary in size and shape. These particles, endowed with motion, combine to make up particular material objects. What we call change is the dissolution of one combination and the appearance of a different one. The particles themselves do not change, but only their combinations. The different properties of the atoms and the differing modes of combination are responsible for the variety of material objects in the universe. In medicine, the phenomena that we call disease, the disturbances which take place in the bodies of sick people, are merely a small subgroup of the phenomena of nature.

This view underwent various modifications during two thousand years or so and reached especial prominence beginning in the seventeenth century. Material particles in eternal motion, combining endlessly, would be the sole ultimate reality, and would enjoy primary status. The actual sensory qualities of things, their properties which we see and hear and feel, had only a secondary or derivative status, and depended on the combination of atoms. The mind, the seat of ideas and perceptions, had a role that was essentially secondary to matter, despite the efforts of philosophers. In its various forms this atomistic view became associated with materialism, and a mechanistic viewpoint.

The second major view, and the one that dominated medicine until the seventeenth century, was the Platonic, especially as modified by Aristotle. Although one school of historians emphasizes the differences between Plato and Aristotle, I belong to the contrary school which, without ignoring the differences, emphasizes the similarities and considers Aristotle as the follower of Plato – a follower in a conceptual as well as a temporal sense.

The Platonic ideas, the 'universals' comprehended by the mind and subsisting eternally, represented not things but rather the properties and relations of things. Particular material objects come into being and pass away, but the universal qualities and relationships that obtain among the particular objects persist. These universals can be discovered by intellectual activity.

This concept was considerably modified by Aristotle. His doctrine of *forms* and of *essences*, existing not by themselves but only in material substrate, embodied Platonic aspects. Aristotle's teachings, much more flexible than Plato's and far better adapted to scientific investigation, found particular application in medicine.

The essence or form involved not merely static qualities but dynamic activity, the 'get up and go' of things, the principles of process and change and development that inhered in things, particularly in living creatures. The concept that dynamic activity made up part of the essence played an important part in biological thinking. Later writers, particularly Galen, emphasized that in living creatures this dynamic activity manifested itself through a series of *faculties*, each of which had a specific power of bringing about a discrete limited goal. Purposeful action and an inherent power of achieving the goal through specific activity, formed a major aspect of the Aristotelian tradition. Aristotelian doctrine was admirably adapted to the study of living creatures which exhibit development and purposive goal activity as part of their existence.

Qualities, forms and essences were the truly real components of the universe. Such a view – I call it the qualitative view of the universe – forms part of a complex intellectual fabric. It stressed the primacy of mind (as contrasted with material particles) and the significance of purpose and goal. It involves a concept of nature as an active process. Nature was an integrating and directing principle, a working together of different parts towards particular goals, and contrasting with blind chance. A corollary of all this is the so-called 'healing power of nature' whereby the drives or faculties of the organism tend toward the restoration of health. Nature had definite trends; and the concept that events happen 'naturally' had real meaning. These various ideas, vague as they were, entered into the doctrine of *vitalism* that played such an important part in medicine. Vitalism gave a central role to mind, purpose, goal, organic wholeness and integrating drives, and contrasted sharply with mechanistic views which might find a place for mind or soul but gave that place but little importance.

In the history of medicine the tensions between the mechanistic and animistic views played an important part and this tension was certainly explicit in Greek philosophy.

The term 'classical heritage' is, of course, extremely broad, and in the present context I restrict myself to a bare mention of philosophical views which shaped the entire course of medical development. Medical history may be regarded as the contrapuntal treatment of such themes as atomism and Platonism, rationalism and empiricism, mechanism and vitalism. In the course of history, sometimes some of these would dominate, sometimes their opposites. In a brief introduction such as this we cannot follow the various convolutions and trends, nor study the reasons for the particular ups and downs, wherein great physicians might adhere to one view or the other, or exhibit a mixture.

In addition to the different metaphysical backgrounds in medical history, there is a separate variable affecting physicians, a property which may be called a critical or analytical sense. By this I mean the capacity physicians may have to examine their own evidence and their own inferences, a concern with the basis on which their assertions rested, and a felt need for proof or demonstration whether through reasoning or sense experience. 'Critical sense' has to do with evidence, validity, proof. We might say that 'critical acumen' revolves around the reaction attributed to Oliver Cromwell: 'By the bowels of Christ, I beseech ye, bethink yourselves that ye may be mistaken.'

The critical physician behaves as if he heeded this injunction. Evidence or reasoning that seemed cogent to one generation could appear extremely inadequate to another. The historian of ideas must try to trace out why one era could accept without questioning the statements, propositions, inferences and beliefs that another era rejected out of hand.

The two most important physicians of antiquity – indeed the two most influential medical figures that ever lived – are Hippocrates and Galen. Hippocrates lived in the golden age of Greece, Galen in the early decline of the Roman Empire. These two men, who lived six centuries apart, are very different one from the other, but each of them brought to medicine much clinical acuity, therapeutic skill, and above all, a sharp critical and analytical attitude. In the excerpts chosen I have tried to show the methods by which Hippocrates and Galen approached the problems of health and disease. The selections will indicate their modes of explanation, the attitudes toward evidence, and the inferences that may be drawn therefrom. Most of what they actually said has been proven incorrect, but this does not in any way affect their stature.

Revolt

The fall of the Roman Empire meant, among other things, a marked shift in the cultural values. Political and social organizations, whose stability had long been wavering, seriously disintegrated. As the cultural patterns broke up, the intellectual components of the culture became dissipated and in large part disappeared from sight. Medicine as a science and an intellectual discipline took part in the disintegration.

During the period of decline, medicine found little encouragement in the West, but as western culture entered into the so-called 'Dark Ages', there occurred a great spurt in the culture of the Arab world. Western knowledge and western medicine – and in our context we can speak particularly of Aristotle and Galen – were introduced into Arabian thought, found there a fertile soil and flourished. Naturally there were modifications under the Arab influence, but the main outlines are recognizable as being derived from western sources.

Among the great Arabian physicians we can mention particularly Rhases (born in 865) and Avicenna (born about 980), who were Persian; while later, in Moslem Spain, Averroes (born 1126) and Maimonides (born 1135) were outstanding. These men, and many of somewhat lesser stature, elaborated and extended medical teachings received from the western world and, while they modified the western components, they created a body of doctrine and of practice that maintained the finest traditions of medicine.

During the Middle Ages, the Arabs not only preserved and extended western medicine but they also were instrumental in reintroducing Greek medicine and much of Greek philosophy back into the western world. With this trend – a sort of reverse flow – we associate particularly the rather shadowy figure of Constantine the African (1020–87), the monastery of Monte

Cassino and the school of Salerno. The transfer of knowledge back from the Arab world took place in the frontier between the two worlds, a frontier centring around the Mediterranean. It is completely fallacious, of course, to think of the Dark Ages as devoid of learning, but the centres of learning were relatively few and the lights burned rather dimly. The interchange with the Arab world did act as a marked impetus.

The great period of medieval culture extended from the eleventh through to the fourteenth centuries, and in its glory rivalled the greatest achievements of the ancient world and the modern world as well. But the institutions and setting were quite different, so much so that we have great difficulty in entering sympathetically into the spirit of the times.

Medieval culture, of which architecture can stand as the vital symbol, reached a very high level. The growth of the universities helped to bring medieval culture to fruition. The reintroduction of Aristotelian philosophy provided new rigor and helped create intellectual patterns of architectonic magnificence, culminating in the scholastic philosophy and the *Summa* of Thomas Aquinas.

The medicine of the medieval period was limited by the intellectual and cultural restrictions that pervaded the era. Largely Hellenic in its theory and oriented to Aristotle in its philosophy, medicine tended to be rationalistic and authoritarian. It depended to a considerable degree on compilation and commentary. Logic played a large role, and there was a tendency to get bogged down in verbalisms. There were two main currents which we may call the *learned* and the *popular*. The learned physician was a highly educated man familiar with the accumulated texts, compilations and commentaries. In the production of such physicians the medical schools of Salerno, Paris, Bologna, Montpellier and Padua were outstanding. But there was also a great deal of popular medicine, practised by those who had little learning. Much of this latter practical medicine was, by later standards, mere superstition, but it did help to keep an empirical orientation that became more and more significant. Important also was the growth of hospitals, principally through church auspices and religious orientation.

Medicine made up an integral part of the medieval civilization, affected by other cultural aspects and in turn reacting on them. The inability of authority and logic to cope with the demands of life affected medicine just as it did the other aspects of medieval activity, and consequently medicine shared in the degeneration that overtook medieval culture. As the whole medieval way of life declined there emerged our modern pattern which developed into its present-day complexity.

The early stages of the transformation from medieval to modern are conventionally called the Renaissance. We cannot answer the question, When was the Renaissance? No longer do we try to give for the transition any precise date, such as 1453 when Constantinople fell. Instead, we recognize a reorientation of interests, a slow transformation of culture that extended roughly from 1300 to 1600. In the latter half of this period we see not so much new currents suddenly emerging as, rather, a development of trends that had been submerged and relatively quiet until they gathered force as external circumstances changed.

Changes occurred in virtually every aspect of medieval civilization. The feudal system, its land economy and the social hierarchy that it produced were breaking up as an economy of trade became more and more prominent. A greater trend to individualism and self expression manifested itself in many different areas, from poetry to geographical exploration. Orientation to this world rather than the other world brought about new attitudes. Dissatisfaction with the church led eventually to the Reformation. The decay of religious institutions and new power politics brought about a new nationalism and changes in political institutions. The changes were many and complex, with deep roots. Some features, such as the invention of printing and the voyages of discovery, are especially dramatic, but they only show to a special degree the property of expansiveness and freedom. There was a reorientation away from the immediate past toward something different. We can, if we wish, think of the Renaissance as revolt against the establishment and we can find more than a few parallels with twentieth-century cultural transformations.

The dissatisfaction with the more immediate past led to two distinct orientations, one more conservative and looking toward the past, the other more radical and looking toward the future. We see this particularly well in medicine where on the one hand was the classical revival that we associate with the term 'humanism', while on the other was adherence to rapidly progressive natural science.

The classical revival that characterized the Renaissance in the late fifteenth and the sixteenth centuries has a clear explanation. The teachings of medieval medicine had depended on the great physicians of antiquity. Classical doctrines, however, were known principally through translations and re-translations, mediated chiefly through Arabic sources and often transformed by Arabic commentators as well as Latin translators. When dissatisfaction arose with one or another aspect of medicine, the physicians tended to blame not the doctrines of the ancients but rather the corrupt state of the texts on which the doctrines rested. If only the original uncorrupted texts could be made available, then perhaps all difficulties could be resolved. Scholars studied the Greek manuscripts of Hippocrates, Galen and others, and translated them into Latin to make them widely available to the medical profession. Among the great physician–scholars eminent as humanists were Thomas Linacre and John Caius.

The humanistic physicians had felt that if they could only recover the original texts of Hippocrates and Galen, then medicine might be more adaptive to changing circumstances. But this hope, that old texts could cast new and effective light, proved vain. The Hellenic heritage had diluted itself in fine-spun distinctions, more and more remote from everyday experience, and even an impeccable text could not satisfy the new demands that the changing environment was producing. Progress did not lie in looking backward.

Another and quite different approach turned its back on the past, which it either expressly rejected or treated with only nominal respect. This forward-looking view broke with tradition, disclaimed the humanistic attitudes and adopted a course that led more directly to modern science. The brilliant advances in Renaissance astronomy, physics and mathematics comprised a trend that competed with humanism and eventually vanquished it.

For the sake of exposition it is convenient to set off the two contrasting views as if they were mutually exclusive alternatives which, between them, applied to all physicians. Such a simplistic and schematic view, however, is quite inaccurate. Major doctrines that have claimed allegiance for many centuries are not instantly overturned. At best, allegiance is loosened in one area, crumbles slightly in another and perhaps vanishes in a third. Various individual changes can nibble away at the framework which have so long supported medical thinking, but do not destroy it. Even the most outspoken medical rebel of the Renaissance, Paracelsus, who so expressly condemned Galen, nevertheless retained a great deal of the Aristotelian background on which Galenic medicine rested. In the Renaissance we can distinguish three groups – the conservatives who retained the older views virtually intact; the radicals who led the assault against the older views; and an intermediate group that tried to combine, somehow, the old and the new.

Medieval medicine, fascinating as it is, did not contribute much to the critical acumen whose development forms the pattern of this book. In the Renaissance, however, there are certain new currents that are crucial to the progress of critical thinking. To illustrate the Renaissance physicians who helped to mould modern medicine, I choose three examples – Vesalius, Paracelsus and Harvey, although Harvey, as a seventeenth-century figure, might be considered post-Renaissance.

These three men represent quite different trends. Vesalius was a man of precision who, devoted to careful observation, showed conclusively that observation took precedence over authority. But Vesalius was not a theorist. He did not try to transform medical theory, not did he intend to revolutionize medical science. He wanted to restore precision and accuracy to medicine and, even though he himself made many errors, he imprinted a wholesome attitude toward facts and empirical observations.

On the other hand, Paracelsus, in his rebellion, was a speculative theorist. He did indeed emphasize observation and he recommended reading the book of nature rather than the writings of Galen. With his empiricism he mingled philosophic speculation that far transcended any experience. He emphasized chemical principles in the study of medicine, but to his chemical insight he occasionally added the antics of a mountebank. He combined mystical and poetical intuition with concrete medical observations. And while he brought new and refreshing currents into medicine, he retained a surprising amount of the Galenic and

Aristotelian thought he affected to despise. Undoubtedly he was one of the most seminal figures in medical history.

Harvey combined all the methodological virtues. A precise observer, a superb experimenter, and a man of productive and yet well-disciplined imagination, he propounded a theory and grounded it so firmly that it achieved the status of fact. His theoretical elaborations stayed close to observation and his inferences remained tied to evidence. The way in which he combined observation and theory illustrates the highest development of critical acumen.

Development

The seventeenth century, to which Harvey really belongs, was an extraordinary period which showed a concentration of genius comparable only to the fifth century BC. Men of surpassing brilliance contributed to literature, art, political science, philosophy, natural science and medicine. At the same time the century was one of turbulence and disorder, punctuated by war and rebellion, revolution and rejection. The key to the era lies, perhaps, in regarding it as the end result of a long transitional period, a transition that had been occurring for two hundred years and reached a climax.

In this process, medicine formed an intrinsic part which we cannot understand without some familiarity with other aspects. Here I can only mention a few strands in the complex fabric.

One major strand was the increasing criticism of rationalism, and the greater dependence on experience. The English took the lead in the empirical revolt, and the names of Francis Bacon and John Locke stand pre-eminent in the history of philosophy.

In the history of medicine, Francis Bacon, a young contemporary of Harvey, is particularly important. He expressly insisted on the importance of sensory experience in philosophy. He demanded that we observe and experiment again and again before we draw facile inferences. And our inferences, derived from our observations, must stand the test of further experience. He appreciated the built-in prejudices and distortions that hindered accurate thinking. These hindrances, drawbacks of our human nature or else produced by our particular environments, must be recognized and counteracted. We must, he insisted, avoid jumping from a few observations to over-arching first principles – the curse of rationalism. Furthermore, Bacon had a sharp sense of the importance of controls. While he himself had only negligible ability in actual investigative technique, he had a high level of critical acumen, and could lay down guidelines that in many ways are still valid today.

Yet while the empirical trend was gathering strength, rationalism continued to flourish. In the first part of the seventeenth century, Descartes was the pre-eminent figure, while later Leibniz maintained the rationalist tradition which his disciples kept vigorous through the entire first half of the eighteenth century.

In the seventeenth- and eighteenth-century context, rationalism meant the reliance on logical analysis, on the processes of inference and deduction from the available data rather than the deliberate search for further data. We commonly speak of 'armchair philosophers' who come to conclusions by using the eye of reason, elaborating concepts and theories whose truth is validated by their rational framework. The mathematician is the best example of the rationalist, and both Descartes and Leibniz were outstanding mathematicians. Rationalism of this type, with admiration for mathematics, was particularly important in late seventeenth-century medical thought, and pervaded much of the eighteenth century.

Of course, neither rationalism nor empiricism are self-subsistent. Each requires the other. We cannot reason without sensory evidence, and we cannot examine experience without some sort of rational framework. It all depends on the relative emphasis. How much of each should we demand? Isaac Newton synthesized reason and experience in a most remarkable manner. A careful observer and experimenter, he embodied the best of the empirical tradition, while as a mathematician he expressed the ideals of rationalism. His scientific methodology, whereby he started with experience and then achieved seemingly universal rules by proper reasoning, stood as the absolute ideal of scientific investigation. The watchword became not experience *or* reason, but experience *and* reason. Investigators who studied various aspects of nature were exhorting each other to find general principles and universal rules (rationalism) but to do so only on the firm basis of experience (empiricism). Unfortunately, while the intent was excellent, the execution was all too often erratic. Experience proved faulty and reason fallacious. The great difficulty was the inadequate critical acumen. Kant, in the next century, helped to combat this lack of a true critical philosophy.

In the medical stream of the latter seventeenth century we must distinguish several quite different currents. In the first part of the century, the Galenic tradition was still supreme. The Galenic physicians, however, faced new discoveries that severely countered the Galenic principles, and adaptation was difficult. Harvey's discovery of the circulation became the cornerstone of the new medicine and eventually contributed markedly to the overturn of Galenism. The new physiology, a powerful force in seventeenth-century medicine, was particularly concerned with the investigation of vessels; and the discovery of the lymphatics as well as the capillaries, lent particular emphasis to concepts of circulation. The blood, and the channels through which it flowed, provided special impetus to so-called humoral theories (although somewhat altered from their original Hippocratic character). The mechanistic physiology of Descartes, which interpreted so much of biological activity in terms of tubes, valves and fluids, strongly supported the hydrodynamic analysis of bodily activities and the role of the humours.

The new physiology was a major component in late seventeenth-century biological thought. A further important influence was the development of microscopy, in which the greatest names are Leeuwenhoek and Hooke. The microscopes, imperfect as they were, opened up to empirical investigation the world of very small objects, too small to be seen with the naked eye, and greatly advanced the actual investigation of biological structure. In addition, such demonstrations gave a great impetus to the atomistic viewpoint, that all things were built out of very minute particles. These ultimate building blocks were, of course, hypothetical. But clearly, when scientists, with the help of appropriate instruments, made visible that which was previously invisible, they gave a greater probability to the reality of atoms. Even though the latter would still be hypothetical, the probability of their existence was increased by what the microscope could reveal.

A further important factor in seventeenth-century medicine was the development of chemistry, in which the names of van

Helmont, Sylvius and Willis were particularly outstanding. The chemists, relying on relatively few experiments, tried to explain biological phenomena in terms quite different from those of the leading physical and mechanical theories. Chemical phenomena, such as the activity of ferments, the interaction of acids and alkalis and the formation of salts with different properties, were considered the basic activities of the living body. Biological processes were interpreted in terms of chemical substances and chemical reactions, rather than in material particles moving in mechanical fashion. But, as with the mechanists, the chemists dealt generally in hypothesis, and built vast superstructures on a skimpy foundation of fact.

The chemists introduced not only important theoretical concepts but practical chemical remedies for disease. Various inorganic substances, metals and salts, might be highly potent agents with pronounced physiological effect. Many physicians eagerly adopted the new chemical remedies and so too did many poorly-trained empirics or quacks, who rebelled against the tight control of the medical establishment.

The many advances in experimental science helped to bring about the triumph of Democritus over Aristotle. The atomistic philosophy, in one guise or another, triumphed over the philosophy of forms and qualities, but the struggle was slow and stubborn. More and more the body came to be regarded as a machine. In this regard the bold physiological speculations of Descartes had enormous influence. He viewed the body as an automaton that obeyed hydraulic and mechanical principles. He distinguished sharply between the soul and the body, and separated off the realm of mind from that of the matter. In this way he felt free to explain physiological processes in mechanistic terms and yet avoided the taint of heresy which a materialistic view of soul would involve.

Another of the most influential seventeenth-century figures was Robert Boyle who, although most famous as a chemist, firmly supported the atomistic philosophy and used the concepts of atomism as explanatory principles in studying natural phenomena. He wrote extensively on biological processes and his voluminous writings are of prime importance in seventeenth-century medicine.

The seventeenth century saw a great improvement in communication, with the foundation of many learned societies which permitted the exchange of ideas among experimenters and theorists. In England the Royal Society had enormous influence, and similar societies on the continent led to a network of communication among the scholars and 'natural philosophers'. These learned societies published various proceedings and transactions, to which physicians and biologists contributed substantially, and which provide invaluable records of contemporary medical investigations.

Of the seventeenth-century medical writers I have, for this anthology, chosen two who represent quite different attitudes and traditions. Thomas Sydenham stands as a model of seventeenth-century empiricism. He paid special attention to the *facts* of observation and indulged only cautiously in inferences based on those facts. Thus he tried to stay close at all times to immediate experience, and although his efforts were by no means always successful, he did give a strong impetus to the empirical movement. He truly deserved the name posthumously bestowed on him, 'The English Hippocrates'. The other selection, from an early work of Friederich Hoffmann, exemplifies the rationalist system-maker, who started with a few basic principles derived from experience. From these principles he created a fairly well integrated system wherein every aspect of experience could be 'explained' by some appropriate part of the logically interlocking framework.

This early book of Hoffmann is quite significant in two ways. It synthesizes many different elements of seventeenth-century medical thought and combines into a single system derivatives from Galenism, the new physiology, the new mechanical concepts, the new chemical ideas. Then it is an excellent transition to the eighteenth century, in which system formation reached a greater elegance and sophistication.

Those factors already clearly visible in the seventeenth century continued to expand and develop in the eighteenth century. Among the systematist–rationalists, the greatest name is Herman Boerhaave, who synthesized into a well-rounded system the most representative portions of contemporary scientific thought. His general leanings were towards the mechanistic viewpoint. And although he was one of the leading chemists of the period, he roundly condemned much of the physiological explanations that the iatrochemists were propounding. In his writings Boerhaave emphasized the prime need for both experience and reason, but despite this, his logical elaboration far outran the factual bases. Nevertheless, he did gather together the various Galenic, mechanical and some of the chemical trends into a well-integrated, satisfying system which avoided the extremes of the more doctrinaire iatromechanists and the iatrochemists. His system was far more polished than that of Hoffmann.

While Boerhaave did not make significant original contributions to medicine, he was probably the most important physician in the first half of the eighteenth century. His synthesis of theories and his general eclecticism provided a widely accepted conceptual background. In addition, he was a skillful clinician and an excellent teacher who drew pupils from all over Europe and even from the New World. For the first half of the eighteenth century he was the most important single medical influence, and his teachings continued, although with diminished influence, for the remainder of the century.

The systematist–rationalist tradition was carried on, in the second half of the century, by William Cullen, who helped to make Scottish medicine the leading force in the medical world and to raise the University of Edinburgh to an eminence that the University of Leiden had enjoyed earlier in the century. Cullen noted the vast array of 'facts' that had accumulated since Boerhaave, and made clear that facts must be organized into a systematic whole. Cullen's system was not as detailed or orderly or logical as Boerhaave's, nor as comprehensive in its explanation force, but it remained in the same tradition.

Cullen achieved considerable fame with his classification of disease (so-called 'nosology'). During the preceding hundred years, great advances in botany and botanical classification had suggested that diseases might be arranged in a way comparable to plants. Although Sydenham had pointed this out in the seventeenth century, little progress was made in classifying diseases until the works of Linnaeus, Sauvages and Cullen. Many later imitators also arranged diseases into classes, genera and species.

The actual nosology, with its ordered arrangement and sub-divisions, is a 'rationalist' activity but there was prior necessity for careful observation and empirical study. Only by observing specific details and scrutinizing empirical characters of disease could students make an analytical classification. The nosological writings of the latter eighteenth century, often based on faulty theory, were quite superficial and they have been frequently ridiculed. But nevertheless the whole movement of nosology provided a stimulus to further empirical development.

John Brown, the most famous of Cullen's pupils, propounded a rationalist system of vague and murky character that neverthe-less was extremely influential for a brief period. Starting with a few facts, Brown elaborated these into an airy conceptual scheme, dealing with 'excitement' and 'excitability' as basic vital prin-ciples. By ignoring vast amounts of 'fact' he was able to throw a false simplicity over medical theory and practice, a simplicity which made considerable appeal among many continental phy-sicians who, at the end of the eighteenth century, were under the influence of the speculative *Naturphilosophie*. John Brown's system also had great influence on Benjamin Rush in the United States.

Despite his brief but vigorous influence, Brown definitely fell outside the main current of medical progress. By the end of the eighteenth century the rationalistic and speculative expositions were in retreat as a new empiricism came to the fore. Yet system-formation continued to have an appeal and in the person of Samuel Hahnemann, founder of homoeopathy, achieved a strong but transitory effect. Hahnemann, who exerted his maximal influence in the second quarter of the nineteenth century, was really an eighteenth-century anachronism who closed his eyes to the medical progress of the latter eighteenth and early nineteenth centuries.

In the latter eighteenth century the systematic–rationalist trend diminished, giving way to the empirical movement which took several different forms. There was a marked upsurge in clinical observation and the reporting of clinical cases and unusual clinical events. A great many of the reports were quite uncritical, but they emphasized the concern with concrete experience rather than theoretical speculation. Increased channels of communication made publication of case reports much more widespread than in the previous century.

In addition, there were many brilliant clinical studies that revealed the highest canons of experimental validity and acumen. Perhaps the most striking of these is the excellent clinical experimentation of James Lind and his studies of scurvy. As is so often the case, military and naval activity have proven the stimulus for considerable advances in medical science and practice. The latter half of the eighteenth century involved military and naval activity that, among the more progressive physicians, promoted careful observation.

A second line of empirical progress had to do with experimental biology rather than medicine as such. The discovery of Abraham Tremblay, who first described the regeneration of the lowly polyp – i.e. the growth of a complete animal from an excised portion – was one of the most significant biological discoveries of the era. In more specifically medical fields the leading experimentalist was perhaps Albrecht Haller who really founded the modern science of physiology. His first text, the *First Lines of Physiology*, published in 1747, was already a substantial advance over the physiological teachings of Boerhaave.

Clinical investigation could be combined with experimental procedures. John Hunter was the outstanding figure in this regard. He combined clinical surgery and medicine with an analytic and experimental trend, a great natural curiosity, and the ability to design and perform relevant experiments which could answer his questions. He had no overall theoretical system and he stands in sharp contrast with the armchair theorist and the rationalist system-maker.

The empirical movement took a somewhat different trend with Morgagni whose careful autopsy dissections showed that, if we want to understand disease, we must have concrete data rather than mere speculation. His careful correlations between the clinical history, physical findings and the autopsy findings served as a model for later pathologists and indicated the significance of the careful postmortem examination.

In the eighteenth century the conflict between the mechanistic and the vitalistic viewpoints reached a new intensity. Descartes had emphasized the similarity between the body of man and the body of animals but pointed out that man alone had a soul. His dualism, while theologically respectable and satisfying, was also a means of eliminating soul from physiological discussions. Unfortunately, there was not a sufficient discrimination between soul and mind, between what today we would consider a theological aspect and a psychological aspect. Descartes regarded animals as machines and denied them any soul. The dualistic philosophy, having given man a soul which animals lacked, differentiated a human from a machine.

From the logical standpoint, it was only a small step to say that man was also a machine, and that the mind of man was not a separate substance but obeyed the same laws that governed machines. La Mettrie took this final step of saying that man also was a machine. He was a speculative thinker and armchair philosopher who, although he plagiarized widely, did have an acute and logical mind. While a tremendous outcry arose against him, he did succeed in placing the 'mind' back into science, and thus helped to unify all of physiology. The indirect result of his doctrine was to separate more firmly than ever the theological aspects of man from the scientific and, so far as physiology is concerned, restored a unity where Descartes had introduced a dualism.

But there had been a strong revolt against crude mechanical views of physiology. George Stahl, in the earlier part of the eighteenth century, vigorously combated the mechanistic tradition. Carrying on the tradition of van Helmont, he utilized the much misunderstood concept of the *anima*. The basic tenet is that living matter differs from dead matter and the behaviour of living matter cannot be explained by reference to tubes, hydrodynamic principles, mechanical motions of particles, friction and the prevalent mechanistic teachings. In emphasizing this viewpoint, Stahl showed critical acumen in stressing observations which the mechanistic views could not readily explain. His doctrines become easier to understand if we interpret the *anima* as an integrating force that somehow combines many discrete individual movements into a well-ordered whole, and that directs behaviour towards definite goals. The concept of anima points to *force* or activity which provides rational interpretation of bodily activity and behaviour. The vitalist emphasized the importance of purpose in understanding living creatures, and any account of behaviour which neglected purpose was deemed unsatisfactory.

Considering the knowledge available at the time, the vitalists certainly showed a much higher degree of critical acumen than did the mechanists. The vitalists, such as Stahl, who regarded the complexity of actual behaviour, were justifiably dissatisfied with the simplistic analysis that the mechanists had furnished. The concept of *anima* is now outmoded and quite hard to grasp, but it did serve as an envelope, covering phenomena that mechanistic views either ignored or explained by unsatisfactory hypotheses.

The concept of an integrating force which tied together many different bodily activities and made them all function toward a common goal proved extremely important in later physiology. The whole doctrine of 'sympathy' was related to this theme, and eventually found a partial explanation in the doctrine of the 'sympathetic' nervous system. While the specific doctrines of Stahl could not hold up under new physiological discoveries (as, for example, the experiments of Tremblay mentioned above), Stahl exerted great influence particularly among the French physicians in Montpellier. Vitalism took on different meanings and the form that Stahl had embraced in turn proved far too simple. But like its opposite, mechanism, eighteenth-century vitalism showed itself quite fertile and eventually merged with its opposite as science advanced. But meanwhile the vitalist movement greatly encouraged critical analysis of mechanistic hypotheses, and provided a stimulus to more careful and precise examination of data and theory.

When we regard the history of medicine as part of the history of ideas and of culture, we see special significance in the decade of the 1740s. In 1740 a quarter century of relative peace came to an end; a period of war and revolution began and continued with only slight interruption for seventy-five years. The deaths of Boerhaave, Hoffmann and Stahl signalled the passing of an old order. Younger men were introducing fresh data and theories. At the same time, political and economic movements, and the resultant social changes, gathered momentum. As the century progressed, the Industrial Revolution brought new wealth. *Mores* changed, as did relative social dominance; new political, social and economic philosophies spread over Europe; the 'Age of Enlightenment' illuminated Europe and America.

The newer trends engendered problems demanding some sort of solution. Social conscience grew stronger and there developed greater concern with public health. The social conscience, helped along by increased wealth, promoted the founding of hospitals. At the same time the inadequacies of traditional medical teaching brought about new orientation: the Scottish universities, for example, began to dominate British medical education; private academies taught certain essentials of medicine; and clinical instruction in hospitals gave practical and realistic direction to medical teaching.

Although political and social theories soared during the 'Age of Reason', medicine became increasingly more sober. An advancing empirical trend of science and philosophy combined to limit speculative rationalism and to smooth the path for further progress.

The French Revolution and the Napoleonic aftermath had a catalytic effect on medicine, bringing about a profound change, but a change more in tempo than in direction. Relatively young men with progressive ideas came to the fore, and their ideas took root more easily than would otherwise have been the case. Observation became more detailed, analysis more precise, discrimination sharper and more critical. Anatomists like Bichat and clinicians like Pinel, Bayle, Laennec or Louis, brought about great progress in clinical observation. They discriminated disease entities, correlated clinical and anatomical findings, and achieved better understanding of disease process. Louis emphasized the quantitative approach to clinical medicine and with his 'numerical method' brought new standards of critical judgement. Yet, with the exception of the stethoscope, which Laennec invented in 1816, the great physicians worked with essentially the same tools that their forebears had used at the end of the seventeenth century. Certainly important advances were being made in chemistry, both organic and inorganic, and in physics, but these advances had little direct impact on medicine.

From the middle of the seventeenth century through the first third of the nineteenth century, medicine did indeed make substantial progress in both practice and theory. Yet these changes proceeded in essentially the same direction. Only toward the middle of the nineteenth century did we see a marked change in direction as new developments in science became translated into new techniques that opened new doors and let men glimpse completely unsuspected vistas. What I call the period of development came to an indefinite end and led gradually to a brilliant flowering in the second half of the nineteenth century.

The selections I have chosen for this development period will illustrate the trends I have mentioned. In the rationalist tradition we have Hoffmann, Boerhaave, Cullen and Hahnemann; in the empirical tradition, Sydenham, Lind, John Hunter and Morgagni. By the turn of the nineteenth century a combination of observation and clinical analysis flourished productively. Bichat and Louis illustrate different phases of this latter movement, while Holmes on the basis of a library study rather than direct personal experience, reveals critical acumen of a high order. The century and a half from Sydenham to Holmes showed a strong development of critical sense. In the next period this critical sense became joined to new techniques and led directly to 'modern' medicine.

Fruition

The first portion of the nineteenth century continued the impulses of the eighteenth and should be considered part of the period of development. Increasing respect for facts and a more critical examination of evidence had crimped the older forms of rationalism and led to flourishing empiricism. In medicine this was a great period of clinical observation and discrimination of clinical entities – a greater concern with what we may call the whole patient. Dogmatism was by no means dead and even maintained considerable popular following, but no longer did unbridled rationalism enjoy the esteem of the best minds. Yet the newer empiricism, flourishing as it was in the early nineteenth century, lacked that ballast which comes only from a sound theory.

Under the flood of new facts and new criticisms, the older eighteenth-century theories disintegrated. In retrospect we can see that a whole new world was opening up, comparable to a bud that matures to a magnificent flower. But while a bud can open relatively quickly, a long period of preparation has preceded the flowering. In nineteenth-century medicine the great breakthrough came when a long series of conceptual advances and technical improvements, stemming largely from chemistry and physics, found an application to medicine. By this time the medical profession had achieved a critical awareness and sophistication appropriate to derive profit from the new tools.

In the 1830s and 1840s a great spurt occurred and led eventually to powerful theories that furnished new conceptual foundations for medicine. I shall mention here only three great areas of advance – microscopy, anaesthesia and microbiology.

Microscopy, although it dates back to the seventeenth century, had made but little progress. The simple microscopes of Leeuwenhoek had fulfilled their maximum capabilities, and the available compound microscopes were too imperfect for productive use. Resolution and definition were not adequate to provide acceptable data, so that alleged observations and descriptions lacked cogency. Microscopy could not furnish objectively valid data that might compel acceptance. Anatomists enlarged their knowledge without the benefit of microscopy. Although Bichat, for example, founded the science of histology, he studied the anatomical and functional characteristics of different tissues without using the microscope.

But by the 1830s the physicists and technologists had solved many of the optical problems that had hindered the development of the microscope. Improved instruments, in the hands of talented observers, made microscopy a truly fruitful science and rendered possible the *cell theory* that quite revolutionized all phases of biology.

In medicine the microscope provided insight into the minute components of the body. Pathologists, studying the innermost nature of disease, carried out investigations wherein new facts permitted the elaboration of new theories. And these theories could be tested with concrete experiments.

A second major innovation was the development of anaesthesia. The immediate humanitarian results were, of course, vast and the control of pain brought about a different attitude towards surgery among patients and surgeons alike. But two other advantages were perhaps even more profound. The control of pain transformed clinical surgery by eliminating the need for speed, permitting tremendous advances in surgical technique, especially when coupled with steps to eliminate infection. Still other advantages accrued to experimental investigators who, particularly in physiology and pathology, could carry out in animals far more complex experiments than were ever before possible. This advance occurred just at a time when new techniques for discrimination, analysis and recording made necessary the control that only anaesthesia could provide.

The third great advance I would mention is in microbiology. The existence of micro-organisms had long been known, but their precise relationship to disease had remained in doubt. Infection and contagion were familiar concepts, although the actual mechanisms of infectious diseases were quite obscure. A series of earnest and brilliant workers provided a new basis for medical practice and medical theory. The isolation of bacteria, the study of their properties, their 'natural history' and their relationships to disease, led to important discoveries. The names of Pasteur, Koch and Lister are particularly famous, but a host of other investigators contributed to the development. A period from about 1870 to approximately 1900 has been called 'the golden age of bacteriology', when important discoveries came in seemingly endless profusion. At the same time the science of immunology had its beginnings, although many decades had to elapse before its own golden age dawned.

The science of epidemiology, already well grounded before the bacteriological era, enjoyed renewed vigour as micro-organisms were identified. Public health and hygiene developed as significant disciplines and assumed importance in the control of many diseases that, in earlier periods, had been quite devastating.

The latter half of the nineteenth century had produced an entire new orientation of medicine, and, indeed, of science in general. The coming of the twentieth century saw advances even more profound. More precise techniques led to unsuspected discoveries and these, in turn, encouraged the production of new techniques which led to further material and conceptual progress. At the same time even closer ties were forged between the disciplines of chemistry and physics and the clinical and investigative aspects of medicine.

Around the turn of the century the discovery of X-rays and

later of radium, the development of precise chemical methods for investigating body fluids, the emergence of specific chemotherapy and the adaptation of electrical methods for studying the heart were a few of the gargantuan steps in medical progress. Studies on metabolism and the discovery of hormones and vitamins welded together the disciplines of physiology, biochemistry and clinical medicine. The identification of so-called 'inborn errors of metabolism' helped to bring medicine into intimate contact with genetics and the broader realm of biology. The vista for progress seemed unlimited. Indeed, the brilliant discoveries of the latter nineteenth century appeared as the merest foretaste of greater wonders to come, and by the third quarter of the twentieth century the promises were undergoing fulfillment.

Medicine, in conjunction with the more rigorous sciences, did indeed accomplish wonders, but certain drawbacks began to appear. There were, for example, the threats of overpopulation and ecologic disaster, as well as social and economic dislocations. These threats are very real, but they fall outside the scope of this volume. More relevant for our purposes is the difficulty in maintaining critical awareness in the face of technological advances. Great discoveries require a sharp critical sense, but if discoveries are to have concrete application in medical practice, practitioners must also have a substantial critical sense. 'Who increaseth knowledge increaseth sorrow', said the preacher, and the sorrow is multiplied if the knowledge is not applied with judgement.

The critical sense had been studied by a long line of philosophers and philosophically orientated scientists. John Stuart Mill, Claude Bernard, Auguste Comte and Robert Koch had all made important contributions and laid a foundation for a modern philosophy of science. But a critical viewpoint in applying knowledge to specific clinical cases lagged behind, and not enough physicians asked themselves the crucial question, 'How sure can I be that I am right?' Reliance on apparatus can obscure critical judgement. In such instances our vaunted medical progress may have only an illusory glitter. Critical judgement is even more important today than in previous centuries when apparatus played no role in medicine.

To illustrate the various advances in the nineteenth and twentieth centuries, I have offered five selections. Virchow, Claude Bernard, Koch, Walter Reed and his associates, and Banting and Best represent towering figures in the history of medicine and also exhibit a splendid scientific methodology. The final selection exemplifies not any great discovery or any particular advance in science but rather the concrete problems that we face when we want to apply our knowledge.

Part One **The Classical Heritage**

from the classical heritage

Hippocrates

Among all physicians throughout the history of medicine the
most revered is undoubtedly Hippocrates, the physician of Cos
who lived in the fifth and fourth centuries BC. Modern scholar-
ship has shown that the writings commonly attributed to Hippocrates were not the work of a single person, but represent a wide
range of doctrines and styles, written by many different individuals over at least 150 years. Some of the so-called Hippocratic
writings were probably the work of the historical Hippocrates,
but for our purposes it is fruitless to dispute over the genuineness
of particular writings. The *Airs, Waters, Places,* is one of those
considered to be genuine. The other text from which we quote,
The Sacred Disease, shows marked differences from the first
and probably was written by a different hand.

The influence of Hippocrates has lasted from the fifth century
BC up to the present time, but during this range of almost 2500
years the significance has changed. Throughout most of this
period the writings of Hippocrates were valued for their substantive content, for the views they gave on the actual diagnosis and
treatment of disease. Today, of course, this aspect has historical
value only. However, at all times, even up to the very present,
the Hippocratic writings have served as a model of method, and
the proper way for a physician to attack the problems of disease.
The first principle is that of precise observation and exact description. Hippocrates had a keen insight into natural phenomena
of disease and provided graphic descriptions which enable us
even today to recognize some of the conditions that he was
describing.

Then, Hippocrates was concerned with treatment. He tried to
identify different kinds of disease, establish sound modes of
treating them, and at the same time avoid speculation.

However, he did not behave like an empiric who based his
remedies on the mere fact that they seemed to work. On the

contrary, Hippocrates sought reasons for the observed phenomena and sequences and, in many of his writings, provided explanations for events and a rationale for the treatments. But in contrast to the speculative thinkers – the philosophers – he did not deal with remote abstractions and fine-spun theories. He gave explanations well within concrete experience, explanations which I call proximal in contrast to those which are remote and speculative. Hippocrates made correlations between different phenomena. In considering that one phenomenon was the 'cause' of another, he utilized certain intermediate explanatory concepts to tie the events together. He relied on the 'humours' or the idea of 'coction', the 'healing power of nature' or a suitable and due 'proportion' among various factors, to explain the causal sequences.

In *Airs, Waters, Places,* Hippocrates indicated the great complexity of the factors relative to disease. He was one of the great ecologists, who pointed out that conditions of health and disease depend on a host of environmental factors. He noted environmental conditions, described physiological and pathological states, and implied a causal connection between them. It is well worthwhile for the reader to note the frequent use of 'and therefore', or 'because', or 'this is due to', or 'owing to' and other terms indicative of causal relationship. Without in any sense suggesting a mono-causational philosophy, he tried to establish correlations between events.

His correlations generally remain on a quite concrete and empirical level. But he also mixed solid observation with rather remote inferences, as in paragraph 14, where he described the heads of the Macrocephali, and then tried to account for them. Along with his 'facts', he worked in the casual statement that 'the seed comes from all parts of the body . . .', as if this were as much a 'fact' of observation as is the bandaging of the head.

It is also worthwhile noting the use that Hippocrates made of controls, as in paragraph 21, where he correlated fertility with bodily habitus and used the slave girls as the controls for the Scythians.

The Sacred Disease maintains the concept that all diseases are part of nature and that the physician must study nature in order to understand disease. Hippocrates provided excellent descriptions of convulsive disorders. He also provided theoretical explanations for the symptoms, but here he removed himself from the field of direct observation and indulged in inference. His terms were those of contemporary physiology – the phlegm, the blood, the brain, the chilling of the blood and the like. But if we ask, 'how did he know that these factors are connected with the disease?', then we find no satisfactory answer. He is in the realm of speculation, even though these speculations are concerned with proximal terms, and not metaphysical entities.

1 Airs, Waters, Places

Excerpts from Hippocrates, 'Airs, Waters, Places', in *The Medical Works of Hippocrates*, translated by John Chadwick and W. N. Mann, Blackwell, 1950, pp. 90–107.

1. Whoever would study medicine aright must learn of the following subjects. First he must consider the effect of each of the seasons of the year and the differences between them. Secondly he must study the warm and the cold winds, both those which are common to every country and those peculiar to a particular locality. Lastly, the effect of water on the health must not be forgotten. Just as it varies in taste and in quality, so does its effect on the body vary as well. When, therefore, a physician comes to a district previously unknown to him, he should consider both its situation and its aspect to the winds. The effect of any town upon the health of its population varies according as it faces north or south, east, or west. This is of the greatest importance. Similarly, the nature of the water supply must be considered; is it marshy and soft, hard as it is when it flows from high and rocky ground, or salty with a hardness which is permanent? Then think of the soil, whether it be bare and waterless or thickly covered with vegetation and well-watered; whether in a hollow and enervating, or exposed and cold. Lastly consider the life of the inhabitants themselves; are they heavy drinkers and eaters and consequently unable to stand fatigue or, being fond of work and exercise, eat wisely but drink sparely?

2. Each of these subjects must be studied. A physician who understands them well, or at least as well as he can, could not fail to observe what diseases are important in a given locality as well as the nature of the inhabitants in general, when he first comes into a district which was unfamiliar to him. Thus he would not be at a loss to treat the diseases to which the inhabitants are liable, nor would he make mistakes as he would certainly do had he not thought about these things beforehand. With the passage of time and the change of the seasons, he would know what epidemics to expect, both in the summer and in the winter, and what particular disadvantages threatened an individual who changed his mode of life. Being familiar with the

progress of the seasons and the dates of rising and setting of the stars, he could foretell the progress of the year. Thus he would know what changes to expect in the weather and, not only would he enjoy good health himself for the most part, but he will be very successful in the practice of medicine. If it should be thought that this is more the business of the meteorologist, then learn that astronomy plays a very important part in medicine since the changes of the seasons produce changes in the mechanism of the body.

3. I shall explain clearly the way in which each of these subjects should be considered. Let us suppose we are dealing with a district which is sheltered from northerly winds but exposed to the warm ones, those, that is, which blow from the quarter between south-east and south-west, and that these are the prevailing winds. Water will be plentiful but it will consist chiefly of brackish surface water, warm in the summer and cold in the winter. The inhabitants of such a place will thus have moist heads full of phlegm, and this, flowing down from the head, is likely to disturb their inner organs. Their constitution will usually be flabby and they tolerate neither food nor drink well. It is a general rule that men with weak heads are not great drinkers because they are particularly liable to hangovers.

The local diseases are these. The women are sickly and liable to vaginal discharges; many of them are sterile, not by nature, but as the result of disease. Miscarriages are common. Children are liable to convulsions and asthma which are regarded as divine visitations and the disease itself as 'sacred'. The men suffer from diarrhoea, dysentery, ague and, in the winter especially, from prolonged fevers. They are also subject to pustular diseases of the skin which are particularly painful at night and also from haemorrhoids. Pleurisy, pneumonia and other acute diseases are rare since such diseases do not flourish in a watery constitution. Moist ophthalmia is not uncommon, but it is neither serious nor of long duration unless an epidemic breaks out owing to some great change in the weather. Catarrh of the head makes those over fifty liable to hemiplegia. They suddenly become 'sunstruck' or cold. Such then are the diseases of the country, except that changes in the weather may produce epidemics in addition.

4. Let us now take the case of a district with the opposite situation, one sheltered from the south but with cold prevailing winds from the quarter between north-west and north-east. The water supply is hard and cold and usually brackish. The inhabitants will therefore be sturdy and lean, tend to constipation, their bowels being intractable, but their chests will move easily. They will be more troubled with bile than with phlegm; they will have hard heads but suffer frequently from abscesses. The special diseases of the locality will be pleurisy and the acute diseases. This is always the case when bellies are hard. Because of this, too, and because they are sinewy, abscesses commonly appear on the slightest pretext. This is also due to their dryness and the coldness of the water. Such men eat with good appetites but they drink little; one cannot both eat and drink a great deal at the same time. Ophthalmia occurs and is of long duration tending to become both serious and chronic, and the eyes suppurate at an early stage. Those under thirty suffer from epistaxis which is serious in summer. Cases of the 'sacred disease' are few but grave. These men live longer than those I described before. Ulcers do not suppurate nor do they spread wildly. Characters are fierce rather than tame. These then are the diseases to which the men of such a district are liable; others only if some change in the weather provokes an epidemic.

The women suffer largely from barrenness owing to the nature of the water; this is hard, permanently so, and cold. Menstruation, too, does not occur satisfactorily but the periods are small and painful. They give birth with difficulty but, nevertheless, miscarriages are rare. After parturition they are unable to feed their babies because the flow of milk is dried up by the intractable hardness of the water. As a result of difficult labour, abscesses and convulsions commonly occur and wasting disease follows. The children suffer from dropsy of the testicles while they are young, but this disappears as they grow up. Puberty is attained late in such a district.

[. . .]

7. [. . .] Now I should like to explain what is the effect of different kinds of water, to indicate which are healthy and which unhealthy, and what effects, both good and bad, they may be expected to produce. Water plays a most important part in

health. Stagnant water from marshes and lakes will necessarily be warm, thick and of an unpleasant smell in summer. Because such water is still and fed by rains, it is evaporated by the hot sun. Thus it is coloured, harmful and bilious-looking. In winter it will be cold, icy and muddied by melting snow and ice. This makes it productive of phlegm and hoarseness. Those who drink it also have large and firm spleens while their bellies are hard, warm and thin. Their shoulders, the parts about the clavicles and their faces are thin too because their spleens dissolve their flesh. Such men have a great appetite for food and drink. Their viscera will be very dry and warm and thus require the stronger drugs. Their spleens remain enlarged summer and winter and, in addition, cases of dropsy are frequent and fatal to a high degree. The reason for this is the occurrence, during the summer, of much dysentery and diarrhoea together with prolonged quartan fevers. Such diseases, when they are of long standing, cause dropsy in people of this type and this proves fatal. These, then, are the summer ailments. In winter, the younger men are liable to pneumonia and to madness. The older men suffer from a fever called *causus* on account of the dryness of their bellies, the women from tumours and leucorrhoea. The latter are weak in the belly and give birth with difficulty. The foetus is large and swollen. During lactation, wasting and pains occur and menstruation does not become properly re-established. The children are specially liable to rupture and the men to varicose veins and ulcers of the legs. People of such nature cannot be long lived and they become prematurely aged. Moreover, sometimes the women appear to have conceived but, when the time of birth approaches, the contents of the belly disappear. This happens when the womb suffers from dropsy. Water which produces these things, I consider harmful in every respect.

We now come to the consideration of water from rock springs. It is hard; either from the soil containing hot waters, or from iron, copper, silver, gold, alum, bitumen or nitre. All these substances are formed by the influence of heat. The water from such ground is bad since it is hard, heating in its effect and causes constipation and dysuria.

The best water comes from high ground and hills covered with earth. This is sweet and clean and, when taken with wine, but little wine is needed to make a palatable drink. Moreover, it is cool in summer and warm in winter because it comes from very deep springs. I particularly recommend water which flows towards the east, and even more that which flows towards the north-east, since it is very sparkling, sweet-smelling and light. Water that is salty, hard and cannot be softened, is not always good to drink. But there are some constitutions and some diseases which benefit by drinking such water and these I shall proceed to detail. The best type of this water is that which comes from springs facing the east. The second best from springs facing the quarter between north-east and north-west, especially the more easterly, and the third from springs between north-west and south-west. The worst is the southern variety, the springs facing between south-west and south-east. These water supplies are worse when the winds are southerly than when they are northerly.

Waters should be used in the following way. A man who is in good and robust health need not distinguish between them, but he may drink whatever is to hand at the moment. But if a sick man wishes to drink what is best for him, he would best regain his health by observing the following rule. If his stomach is hard and liable to become inflamed, the sweetest, lightest and most sparkling water is best for him; but if his stomach is soft, moist and full of phlegm, the hardest and saltiest are best since these will best dry it up. The water that is best for cooking and softest is likely to relax and soften the stomach. Hard water that is not softened by boiling tends to make the stomach contract and dries it up. Owing to ignorance, there is a general fallacy about brackish water. Salty water is thought to be a laxative; actually the opposite is the case and permanently hard water tends to make the bowels costive.

8. We now pass from spring water to a consideration of rain water and water from snow. Rain water is very sweet, very light and also very fine and sparkling since the sun, drawing it up, naturally seizes upon the finest and lightest water, as is proved by the salt which is left behind. The brine is left on account of its thickness and heaviness and becomes salt, but the sun draws up the finest elements because of their lightness. It draws it up not only from ponds, but also from the sea and in fact from any source which contains moisture; there is nothing

that does not contain some. Even from human beings, it draws off the finest and lightest part of the body's humours. A very good proof of this is seen when a man goes and sits in the sun wearing a cloak. Where sunlight falls on the body, no sweat will be seen, but the part which is shaded or protected by something becomes damp with sweat. This is because the sun draws up the sweat and makes away with it; but where the body is shaded, the sweat remains because the sunlight cannot get at it. If the man goes in the shade, the whole body sweats alike because the sun is no longer on him. Rain water, being composed of a mixture of so many elements, quickly becomes rotten on standing and exhales a foul smell. But when it has been drawn up into the air, it travels round and mixes with the air; the dark and cloudy part is separated and becomes cloud and mist, while the clearest and lightest part is left, sweetened by the sun heating and boiling it. Everything is sweetened by boiling. So long as it is scattered and does not mass together, it remains floating in the air. But when it is gathered and collected suddenly by the assault of contrary winds, then it falls wherever there happens to be the densest cloud. This is most likely to happen when a wind has gathered some clouds together and is driving them along and then another wind suddenly confronts it with another mass of clouds. Then the first cloud is stopped and the following ones pile up on it till it becomes thick and black and dense, and its weight causes it to turn to rain and fall. Rain water, therefore, is likely to be the best of all water, but it needs to be boiled and purified. If not, it has a foul smell and causes hoarseness and deepness of the voice in those that drink it.

Water from snow and ice is always harmful because, once it has been frozen, it never regains its previous quality. The light, sweet and sparkling part of it is separated and vanishes leaving only the muddiest and heaviest part. You may prove this, if you wish, by measuring some water into a jar and then leaving it out in the open air on a winter's night in the coldest spot you can find. Next morning bring it back into the warmth again and, when it has thawed, measure it a second time. You will find the quantity considerably less. This shows that in the process of freezing, the lightest and finest part has been dried up and lost, for the heaviest and densest part could not disappear thus. For this reason I consider such water to be the most harmful for all purposes.

9. The effect of drinking water collected from many different sources, that is, from large rivers fed by smaller streams and from lakes into which many streams flow from different directions, is to cause a propensity to stone, gravel in the kidneys, strangury, pain in the loins and rupture. The same is true of water brought long distances from its source. The reason for this is that no two sorts of water can be alike but some will be sweet, some salt and astringent and some from warm springs. When they are all mixed they quarrel with one another and the strongest is always the dominant. But each one has not always the same strength and sometimes one is dominant, sometimes another according to which wind is blowing. One will be made strong by the north wind, another by the south and so on. Such water will leave a sediment of sand and slime at the bottom of the jar and it is by drinking this that the diseases mentioned above are caused. There are, however, certain exceptions and these I shall detail.

Those whose stomachs are healthy and regular, and whose bladders are not subject to inflammation, nor in whom the neck of the bladder is overmuch obstructed, pass water easily and nothing collects in the bladder. But if the belly is liable to fever the same must be true of the bladder, and when this organ is heated with fever, the neck of the bladder becomes inflamed and does not allow the urine to pass which instead becomes heated and condensed. The finest and clearest part is separated, passes through and is voided. The densest and cloudiest part is gathered together and precipitates in small pieces at first and then in larger ones. The gravel formed is rolled round by the urine and coalesces to form a stone. When water is passed this falls over the neck of the bladder, and being pressed down by the pressure of the urine, prevents the urine from being passed. Great pain is thus caused. As a result, children suffering from stone rub or pull at their private parts because they think that in them lies the cause why they cannot make water. The fact that people who suffer from stone have very clear urine is proof that the densest and muddiest part remains in the bladder and collects there. This is the explanation of most cases of this disease but, in children, stones may also be caused by milk. If milk is not healthy but too warm and bilious-looking, it heats the stomach and the bladder and the urine is heated and a similar result is produced to that already described. Indeed, I assert that it is better to give children wine watered down as much as possible for this neither burns the veins nor dries them up too much. Female children are less liable to stone because the urethra is short and wide and the urine is passed easily. Neither do they masturbate as the males do, nor touch the urethra. In the female the urethra is short; in males it is not straight and it is narrow as well. Moreover, girls drink more than boys.

10. Now let us consider the seasons and the way we can predict whether it is going to be a healthy or an unhealthy year.

[. . .]

If the winter is wet and mild with southerly winds and this is followed by a wintry dry spring with the wind in the north, the effect will be as follows. First, women who happen to be pregnant and approaching term in the spring are likely to have miscarriages. Or, if they do give birth, the babies are so weak and sickly that either they die at once or, if they survive, they are frail and weak and very liable to disease. The men are liable to dysentery and dry ophthalmia, while some will suffer from catarrh of the head which may spread to the lungs. It is those who are full of phlegm, as well as the women, who are likely to suffer from dysentery since the phlegm flows down from the brain on account of their moist constitutions. On the other hand, those who are full of bile suffer from dry ophthalmia on account of the warmth and dryness of the flesh, while the old, owing to the permeability and exhaustion of the blood vessels, suffer from catarrh. This last illness may prove suddenly fatal to some, while others are afflicted with a right- or left-sided hemiplegia. The explanation of these diseases is this. When the winter is warm with wet south winds, neither the brain nor the blood vessels become consolidated. Thus, when spring comes with dry cold northerly winds, the brain becomes stiff and cold just when it ought to thaw and become purified by running of the nose and hoarseness. It is the sudden change when the heat of summer comes that is responsible for these diseases.

[. . .]

12. I now want to show how different in all respects are Asia

and Europe, and why races are dissimilar, showing individual physical characteristics. It would take too long to discuss this subject in its entirety but I will take what seem to me to be the most important points of difference.

Asia differs very much from Europe in the nature of everything that grows there, vegetable or human. Everything grows much bigger and finer in Asia, and the nature of the land is tamer, while the character of the inhabitants is milder and less passionate. The reason for this is the equable blending of the climate for it lies in the midst of the sunrise facing the dawn. It is thus removed from extremes of heat and cold. Luxuriance and ease of cultivation are to be found most often when there are no violent extremes, but when a temperate climate prevails. All parts of Asia are not alike, but that which is centrally placed between the hot and the cold parts is the most fertile and well wooded; it has the best weather and the best water, both rain water and water from springs. It is not too much burnt up by the heat nor dessicated by parching drought; it is neither racked by cold nor drenched by frequent rains from the south or by snow. Crops are likely to be large, both those which are from seed and those which the earth produces of her own accord. But as the fruits of the latter are eaten by man, they have cultivated them by transplanting. The cattle raised there are most likely to do well, being most prolific and best at rearing their young. Likewise, the men are well made, large and with good physique. They differ little among themselves in size and physical development. Such a land resembles the spring time in its character and the mildness of the climate.

[. . .]

14. I will leave out the minor distinctions of the various races and confine myself to the major differences in character and custom which obtain among them. First the Macrocephali; no other race has heads like theirs. The chief cause of the length of their heads was at first found to be in their customs, but nowadays nature collaborates with tradition and they consider those with the longest heads the most nobly born. The custom was to mould the head of the newly-born children with their hands and to force it to increase in length by the application of bandages and other devices which destroy the spherical shape of the head and produce elongation instead. The characteristic was thus acquired

at first by artificial means, but, as time passed, it became an inherited characteristic and the practice was no longer necessary. The seed comes from all parts of the body, healthy from the healthy parts and sickly from the sickly. If therefore bald parents usually have bald children, grey-eyed parents grey-eyed children, if squinting parents have squinting children, why should not long-headed parents have long-headed children? The custom of binding the head has also become obsolete through intercourse with other peoples.

[. . .]

17. In Europe, on the other hand, and living round Lake Maeotis, there is a special race of Scythians which differs from all other peoples. They go by the name of Sauromatae. Their women ride horses and shoot arrows and hurl javelins from the saddle and they fight in campaigns as long as they remain virgins. Nor do they lose their virginity until they have killed three of their enemies and have offered such sacrifices as are prescribed by ritual law. But once a woman has taken to herself a husband she does not ride again unless military necessity should require their total forces to take to the field. The women have no right breast since their mothers heat a specially made iron and apply it to the breast while they are still children. This prevents the breast from growing and all the strength and size of it goes into the right arm and shoulder instead.

18. As regards the appearances of other tribes of Scythians, the same is true of them as is true of the Egyptians, namely, that they have certain racial characteristics, but differ little among themselves. They differ, however, from the Egyptians in that their peculiarities are due to cold instead of to heat. The so-called Scythian desert is a grassy plain devoid of trees and moderately watered, for there are large rivers there which drain the water from the plains. Here live the Scythians who are called nomads because they do not live in houses but in wagons. The lighter wagons have four wheels but some have six, and they are fenced about with felt. They are built like houses, some with two divisions and some with three, and they are proof against rain, snow and wind. The wagons are drawn by two or three yokes of hornless oxen: hornless because of the cold. The women live in these wagons while the men ride on horseback, and they are followed

by what herds they have, oxen and horses. They stay in the same place as long as there is enough grass for the animals but as soon as it fails they move to fresh ground. They eat boiled meat and drink the milk of mares from which they also make a cheese.

19. So much then for their mode of life and customs. As regards their physical peculiarities and the climate of their lands, the Scythian race is as far removed from the rest of mankind as can be imagined and, like the Egyptians, they are all similar to one another. They are the least prolific of all peoples and the country contains very few wild animals and what there are are very small. [. . .] Northerly winds, chilled with snow and ice and charged with great rains, blow continuously and never leave the mountains which makes them most inhospitable. During the daytime, mist often covers the plains where the people live and, in fact, winter is nearly continuous all the year round. [. . .] The people differ little in physique as they always eat similar food, wear the same clothes winter and summer, breathe moist thick air, drink water from snow and ice and do no hard work. The body cannot become hardened where there are such small variations in climate; the mind, too, becomes sluggish. For these reasons their bodies are heavy and fleshy, their joints are covered, they are watery and relaxed. The cavities of their bodies are extremely moist, especially the belly, since, in a country of such a nature and under such climatic conditions, the bowels cannot be dry. All the men are fat and hairless and likewise all the women, and the two sexes resemble one another. Owing to the lack of variation in the weather, there is no interference with the coagulation of the semen unless there is some intercurrent disease.

20. As a proof of this moistness of the constitution, I may instance the following. You will find that the majority of the Scythians, especially those who are nomads, are cauterized on the shoulders, arms, wrists, chests, hips and loins. This is done simply for the softness and moistness of their constitutions because otherwise they could neither bend their bows nor put any weight into throwing the javelin. But when they have been cauterized the moisture is dried out of their joints and their bodies become more sinewy and stronger and their joints may then be seen. They grow up flabby and stout for two reasons. First because

they are not wrapped in swaddling clothes, as in Egypt, nor are they accustomed to horse-riding as children, which makes for a good figure. Secondly, they sit about too much. The male children, until they are old enough to ride, spend most of their time sitting in the wagons and they walk very little since they are so often changing their place of residence. The girls get amazingly flabby and podgy. The Scythians have ruddy complexions on account of the cold, for the sun does not burn fiercely there. But the cold causes their fair skins to be burnt and reddened.

21. People of such constitution cannot be prolific. The men lack sexual desire because they are so flabby and because of the softness and coldness of their bellies, a condition which least inclines men to intercourse. Moreover, being perpetually worn out with riding they are weak in the sexual act when they do have intercourse. These reasons suffice as far as the men are concerned. In the case of the women, fatness and flabbiness are also to blame. The womb is unable to receive the semen and they menstruate infrequently and little. The opening of the womb is sealed by fat and does not permit insemination. The women, being fat, are easily tired and their bellies are cold and soft. Under such conditions it is impossible for the Scythians to be a prolific race. As a good proof of the sort of physical characteristics which are favourable to conception, consider the case of serving wenches. No sooner do they have intercourse with a man than they become pregnant, on account of their sturdy physique and their leanness of flesh.

2 The Sacred Disease

Excerpts from 'The Sacred Disease', in *The Medical Works of Hippocrates*, translated by John Chadwick and W. N. Mann, Blackwell, 1950, pp. 179–89.

1. I do not believe that the 'Sacred Disease' is any more divine or sacred than any other disease but, on the contrary, has specific characteristics and a definite cause. Nevertheless, because it is completely different from other diseases, it has been regarded as a divine visitation by those who, being only human, view it with ignorance and astonishment. This theory of divine origin, though supported by the difficulty of understanding the malady, is weakened by the simplicity of the cure consisting merely of ritual purification and incantation. If remarkable features in a malady were evidence of divine visitation, then there would be many 'sacred diseases'. Quotidian, tertian and quartan fevers are among other diseases no less remarkable and portentous and yet no one regards them as having a divine origin. I do not believe that these diseases have any less claim to be caused by a god than the so-called 'sacred' disease but they are not the objects of popular wonder. Again, no less remarkably, I have seen men go mad and become delirious for no obvious reason and do many strange things. I have seen many cases of people groaning and shouting in their sleep, some who choke; others jump from their bed and run outside and remain out of their mind till they wake, when they are as healthy and sane as they were before, although perhaps rather pale and weak. These things are not isolated events but frequent occurrences. There are many other remarkable afflictions of various sorts, but it would take too long to describe them in detail.

2. It is my opinion that those who first called this disease 'sacred' were the sort of people we now call witch-doctors, faith-healers, quacks and charlatans. These are exactly the people who pretend to be very pious and to be particularly wise. By invoking a divine element they were able to screen their own failure to give suitable treatment and so called this a 'sacred' malady to conceal their ignorance of its nature. By picking their phrases carefully, prescribing purifications and incantations

along with abstinence from baths and from many foods unsuitable for the sick, they ensured that their therapeutic measures were safe for themselves. The following fish were forbidden as being the most harmful: mullet, black-tail, hammer and eel. Goat, venison, pork and dog were considered most likely among meats to upset the stomach. Of fowls: cock, turtle-dove and buzzard and those which are considered very rich were forbidden; white mint, garlic and onion were excluded from the diet because over-flavoured food is not good for a sick man. Further, their patients were forbidden to wear black because it is a sign of death, to use goat-skin blankets or to wear goat-skins, nor were they allowed to put one foot on the other or one hand on the other; and all these things were regarded as preventative measures against the disease. These prohibitions are added on account of the divine element in the malady, suggesting that these practitioners had special knowledge. They also employ other pretexts so that, if the patient be cured, their reputation for cleverness is enhanced while, if he dies, they can excuse themselves by explaining that the gods are to blame while they themselves did nothing wrong; that they did not prescribe the taking of any medicine whether liquid or solid, nor any baths which might have been responsible.

I suppose none of the inhabitants of the interior of Libya can possibly be healthy seeing that they sleep on goat skins and eat goat meat. In fact, they possess neither blanket, garment nor shoe that is not made of goat skin, because goats are the only animals they keep. If contact with or eating of this animal causes the disease while abstinence from it cures the disease, then diet is alone the factor which decides the onset of the disease and its cure. No god can be blamed and the purifications are useless and the idea of divine intervention comes to nought.

3. It seems, then, that those who attempt to cure disease by this sort of treatment do not really consider the maladies thus treated of sacred or of divine origin. If the disease can be cured by purification and similar treatment then what is to prevent its being brought on by like devices? The man who can get rid of a disease by his magic could equally well bring it on; again there is nothing divine about this but a human element is involved. By such claims and trickery, these practitioners pretend a deeper

knowledge than is given to others; with their prescriptions of 'sanctifications' and 'purifications', their patter about divine visitation and possession by devils, they seek to deceive. And yet I believe that all these professions of piety are really more like impiety and a denial of the existence of the gods, and all their religion and talk of divine visitation is an impious fraud which I shall proceed to expose.

[. . .]

5. I believe that this disease is not in the least more divine than any other but has the same nature as other diseases and a similar cause. Moreover, it can be cured no less than other diseases so long as it has not become inveterate and too powerful for the drugs which are given.

Like other diseases it is hereditary. If a phlegmatic child is born of a phlegmatic parent, a bilious child of a bilious parent, a consumptive child of a consumptive parent and a splenetic child of a splenetic parent, why should the children of a father or mother who is afflicted with this disease not suffer similarly? The seed comes from all parts of the body; it is healthy when it comes from healthy parts, diseased when it comes from diseased parts. Another important proof that this disease is no more divine than any other lies in the fact that the phlegmatic are constitutionally liable to it while the bilious escape. If its origin were divine, all types would be affected alike without this particular distinction.

6. So far from this being the case, the brain is the seat of this disease, as it is of other very violent diseases. I shall explain clearly the manner in which it comes about and the reason for it.

The human brain, as in the case of all other animals, is double; a thin membrane runs down the middle and divides it. This is the reason why headache is not always located in the same site but may be on either side or, sometimes, affects the whole head. There are a large number of tenuous veins which extend to this structure from all parts of the body; there are also two large vessels, one coming from the liver and one from the spleen. That which comes from the liver is disposed as follows: one half runs down on the right side in relation with the kidney and the lumbar muscles, to reach the inside of the thigh and thence continues to the foot. It is called the 'hollow vein'. The other half courses upwards through the right side of the diaphragm and lies close to the right lung; branches split off to the heart and to the right arm while the remainder passes up behind the clavicle on the right side of the neck and there lies subcutaneously so as to be visible. It disappears close to the ear and then divides; the larger part finishes in the brain while smaller branches go separately to the right ear, the right eye and to the nostril. Such is the distribution of the blood vessels from the liver. There is also a vein which extends both upwards and downwards from the spleen on the left side of the body; it is similar to that coming from the liver but is thinner and weaker.

7. It is through these blood-vessels that we respire, for they allow the body to breathe by absorbing air, and it is distributed throughout the body by means of the minor vessels. The air is cooled in the blood-vessels and then released. Air cannot remain still but must move; if it remains still and is left behind in some part of the body, then that part becomes powerless. A proof of this is that if we compress some of the smaller blood-vessels when we are lying or sitting down, so that air cannot pass through the vessels, then numbness occurs at once. Such, then, is the nature of blood-vessels.

8. Now this disease attacks the phlegmatic but not the bilious. Its inception is even while the child is still within its mother's womb, for the brain is rid of undesirable matter and brought to full development, like the other parts, before birth. If this 'cleansing' takes place well and moderately so that neither too much nor too little comes away, the head is most healthy. But if there is too much lost from the whole brain so that a lot of wasting occurs, the head will be feeble and, when the child grows up, he will suffer from noises in the head and be unable to stand the sun or the cold. If the discharge is excessive from one part only, such as an eye or an ear, or one blood-vessel becomes shrivelled up, then whichever part be wasted in that way becomes damaged. On the other hand, if this 'cleansing' does not take place but the material is retained in the brain, a phlegmatic constitution is bound to result.

Sometimes phlegm, which should have been purged out during life in the womb, remains during early life and is only got rid of in the later years. This is what happens in the case of children who suffer from ulcers of the head, ears and flesh, and who salivate and discharge mucus; they get better as they grow older. Those who have been purged of the phlegm in this way are not troubled by this disease, but for those who have neither been purged in this way by ulceration and discharges of mucus and saliva, nor have been purged in the womb, it is most dangerous to be attacked with it.

9. If these discharges should make their way to the heart, the chest is attacked and palpitation or asthma supervenes; some patients even become kyphotic. For when cold mucus reaches the lungs and heart, the blood is chilled and the blood-vessels, as a result of being violently cooled in the region of the lungs and heart, jump and the heart palpitates. Such circumstances force the onset of asthma and diseases characterized by orthopnoea because, until the mucus which has flowed down has been warmed and dissipated by the blood-vessels, it is impossible to inspire as much air as is needed. When the phlegm has been removed, palpitation and asthma stop. The length of an attack depends upon the quantity of mucus which has flowed in. The more frequent these discharges of mucus, the more frequent the attacks. These effects, however, occur only if the discharge makes its way to the lungs and heart; if it reaches the stomach, diarrhoea results.

10. Should these routes for the passage of phlegm from the brain be blocked, the discharge enters the blood-vessels which I have described. This causes aphonia, choking, foaming at the mouth, clenching of the teeth and convulsive movements of the hands; the eyes are fixed, the patient becomes unconscious and, in some cases, passes a stool. I will explain the reason for each of these signs. Loss of voice occurs when the phlegm suddenly descends in the blood-vessels and blocks them so that air can pass neither to the brain nor to the hollow blood-vessels nor to the body cavities, and thereby inhibits respiration. For when a man draws in breath through the mouth and nose, the air passes first to the brain and then the greater part goes to the stomach, but some flows into the lungs and blood-vessels. From these places it is dispensed throughout the rest of the body by means of the blood-vessels. The air which flows into the stomach cools it but makes no other contribution. But that which goes to the lungs and

blood-vessels thence enters the body cavities and the brain and has a further purpose. It induces intelligence and is necessary for the movement of the limbs. Therefore, when the blood-vessels are shut off from this supply of air by the accumulation of phlegm and thus cannot afford it passage, the patient loses his voice and his wits. The hands become powerless and move convulsively for the blood can no longer maintain its customary flow. Divergence of the eyes takes place when the smaller blood-vessels supplying them are shut off and no longer provide an air supply; the vessels then pulsate. The froth which appears at the lips comes from the lungs for, when air no longer enters them, they produce froth which is expectorated as in the dying. The violence of choking causes the passage of stools; choking is caused by the liver and the thoracic contents compressing the diaphragm and thus obstructing the entry into the stomach. This action results from the amount of air taken in by the mouth being less than normal. When air is shut off in the vessels of the limbs and cannot escape owing to the obstruction of the vessels with phlegm, it moves violently up and down through the blood and the convulsions and pain thus caused produce the kicking movements.

All these symptoms are produced when cold phlegm is discharged into the blood which is warm, so chilling the blood and obstructing its flow. If the cold material is copious and thick, the result is immediately fatal as though its coldness had overcome and destroyed the blood. If the quantity is less, however, although at first it may have the upper hand and obstruct respiration, in the end it is dispersed throughout the blood which is plentiful and warm, and if it be overcome in this way, the blood-vessels again take in air and consciousness returns.

11. Infants who suffer from this disease usually die if the phlegm is copious and if the weather is southerly. Their little blood-vessels are too narrow to absorb a large quantity of inspissated phlegm and so the blood is at once chilled and frozen, thus causing death. If the amount of phlegm is small and enters both main vessels, or if it enters but one of them, the patient survives but bears the stigmata. Thus the mouth may be distorted, or an eye, a hand or the neck; according to the part of the body in which some blood-vessel became filled and obstructed with phlegm and thus rendered inadequate. As a result of this

damage to the blood-vessel, the corresponding part of the body must necessarily be weakened.

[. . .]

12. Adults neither die from an attack of this disease, nor does it leave them with palsy. The blood-vessels in patients of this age are capacious and full of hot blood; as a result, the phlegm cannot gain the upper hand and chill and freeze the blood. Instead the phlegm is quickly overcome as it is diluted by the blood, and the vessels take in air again so that consciousness returns and the symptoms mentioned above are less pronounced owing to the strength of the patient.

[. . .]

14. When the disease has been present from childhood, a habit develops of attacks occurring at any change of wind and specially when it is southerly. This is hard to cure because the brain has become more moist than normal and is flooded with phlegm. This renders discharges more frequent. The phlegm can no longer be completely separated out; neither can the brain, which remains wet and soaked, be dried up. This observation results specially from a study of animals, particularly of goats which are liable to this disease. Indeed, they are peculiarly susceptible to it. If you cut open the head you will find that the brain is wet, full of fluid and foul-smelling, convincing proof that disease and not the deity is harming the body. It is just the same with man, for when the malady becomes chronic, it becomes incurable. The brain is dissolved by phlegm and liquefies; the melted substance thus formed turns into water which surrounds the brain on the outside and washes round it like the sea round an island. Consequently, fits become more frequent and require less to cause them. The disease therefore becomes very chronic as the fluid surrounding the brain is dilute because its quantity is so great, and as a result it may be quickly overcome by the blood and warmed.

15. Patients who suffer from this disease have a premonitory indication of an attack. In such circumstances they avoid company, going home if they are near enough, or to the loneliest spot they can find if they are not, so that as few peoples as possible will see them fall, and they at once wrap their heads up in their coats. This is the normal reaction to embarrassment

and not, as most people suppose, from fear of the demon. Small children, from inexperience and being unaccustomed to the disease, at first fall down wherever they happen to be. Later, after a number of attacks, they run to their mothers or to someone whom they know well when they feel one coming on. This is through fear and fright at what they feel, for they have not yet learnt to feel ashamed.

Galen

Galen was probably the most influential physician that ever lived, for his doctrines held virtually complete sway over western medicine for almost 1400 years, and only in the seventeenth century did these teachings crumble, to be replaced by other doctrines and other systems. The teachings of Galen are extremely complex, and only a relatively small part has been translated into English. For the present volume we can provide merely a glimpse of the Galenic principles, and we will emphasize the methodological aspects, with only a few references to the substantive content.

The essence of Galenic teaching may be summarized in the single word 'dynamism'. He saw nature as an active force with a coherent integrated purposeful activity that the physician must try to understand. To make the process intelligible, Galen devised a special vocabulary. Observed phenomena he identified as 'effects', which derive from activities. Activity involves change, and he equated change with motion. The cause of the motion – i.e., the cause of the activity – he called a faculty.

Galen's writings are essentially descriptive. In his investigations of nature he tried to identify and isolate various phenomena and break them up into their component parts, each of which, in turn, was a phenomenon to be described. Thus, under the term 'natural faculties' he considered various processes which we identify with growth, digestion, metabolism. In the category of growth, for example, it is necessary first to describe the growth of the embryo. How does it happen that from an undifferentiated mass there develops a highly differentiated organism, with many different tissues? The various degrees of differentiation he considered to result from specific dynamic processes. The nature of the process was unknown to him but he postulated a cause or 'faculty', consistent with the dominant Aristotelian metaphysics.

By indicating that a particular change was due to a 'faculty' he accomplished two tasks. First, he defined a specific process, distinct from other processes. In other words, by analysing complex vital phenomena he could break them down into specific steps. Then, he indicated that each of these steps was due to a specific functional activity, the 'faculty'. This nomenclature may seem to us only a tautology, but such a judgement is not quite fair. Galen was pointing to some inner essential force that brought about a specific process. Differently stated, a particular effect was not a general or non-specific by-product but a specific, orderly chain of events, rooted in the inner nature of things. The faculty was intimately related to the inner essence, and may be construed as representing the Form, in the Aristotelian sense, of the phenomenon. The Form was the controlling force which directed the process toward a specific end.

The concept of end or goal is central to Galenic thought. Galen could perceive a purpose in everything, and every structure, every activity, existed for a purpose. Function and structure were intimately connected and reason could yield an answer regarding the purpose of a particular structure.

Galen was a firm rationalist, who used logic to prove his points. For example, when considering the function of the kidneys, he set out various logical alternatives, with the supposition that these alternatives were, between them, completely exhaustive with no possibilities left out of account. Then, taking each of the alternatives in turn, he showed that each was untenable – it might be contrary to observed fact, or involve a logical contradiction with some previously accepted teaching. When the various alternatives had been eliminated, what remained was necessarily true by exclusion. This mode of reasoning might be satisfactory in certain aspects of mathematics, where the alternatives could be demonstrated to be jointly exhaustive, with no ground left over. But in empirical matters Galen could not prove that there was no middle ground left over.

We see a splendid example of this methodology when he considered the way in which urine was excreted. Galen's 'proof' that excretion of urine takes place through 'attraction' has considerable force if we assume that there is no circulation. But the entire force depends on the supposition that there is no circulation. Once we bring in the possibility that the blood circulates, then his entire logical apparatus falls to the ground.

But we must not ignore the fact that Galen, in addition to being an acute logician, was also an excellent experimenter. The experiments that he designed to show that the urine in the bladder comes from the kidneys, are indeed well planned and cogent.

We also see that Galen was a polemicist, fond of disputing, and quite abusive to his opponents. Much of what we know about the earlier physicians comes from the accounts that he gave, preparatory to refuting them.

The study of Galen is rewarding, not only for the insight it gives into the workings of a great mind, but as a preparation for understanding the changes that took place in sixteenth- and seventeenth-century medicine.

3 On the Natural Faculties

Excerpts from Galen, *On the Natural Faculties*, translated by Arthur
John Brock, Heinemann, 1952 and Harvard University Press, pp. 3–113.

Book I

II [. . .]

The discussion which follows we shall devote entirely [. . .] to
an inquiry into the number and character of the *faculties* of
nature, and what is the effect which each naturally produces.
Now, of course, I mean by an effect that which has already come
into existence and has been completed by the *activity* of these
faculties – for example, blood, flesh, or nerve. And *activity* is the
name I give to the active change or *motion*, and the *cause* of this
I call a *faculty*. Thus, when food turns into blood, the motion of
the food is passive, and that of the vein active. Similarly, when
the limbs have their position altered, it is the muscle which
produces, and the bones which undergo the motion. In these
cases I call the motion of the vein and of the muscle an *activity*,
and that of the food and the bones a *symptom* or *affection*, since
the first group undergoes *alteration* and the second group is
merely *transported*. One might, therefore, also speak of the
activity as an *effect* of nature – for example, digestion, absorption,
blood-production.

[. . .]

IV [. . .] So long as we are ignorant of the true essence of the
cause which is operating, we call it a *faculty*. Thus we say that
there exists in the veins a blood-making faculty, as also a digestive
faculty in the stomach, a pulsatile faculty in the heart, and in
each of the other parts a special faculty corresponding to the
function or activity of that part. If, therefore, we are to investigate
methodically the number and kinds of faculties, we must begin
with the effects; for each of these effects comes from a certain
activity, and each of these again is preceded by a cause.

V The effects of nature, then, while the animal is still being
formed in the womb, are all the different *parts* of its body, and
after it has been born, an effect in which all parts share is the

progress of each to its full size, and thereafter its maintenance of itself as long as possible.

The activities corresponding to the three effects mentioned are necessarily three – one to each – namely, genesis, growth and nutrition. Genesis, however, is not a simple activity of nature, but is compounded of *alteration* and of *shaping*. That is to say, in order that bone, nerve, veins and all other [tissues] may come into existence, the *underlying substance* from which the animal springs must be *altered*; and in order that the substance so altered may acquire its appropriate shape and position, its cavities, out-growths, attachments, and so forth, it has to undergo a *shaping* or *formative* process. One would be justified in calling this substance which undergoes alteration the *material* of the animal, just as wood is the material of a ship, and wax of an image.

Growth is an increase and expansion in length, breadth, and thickness of the solid parts of the animal (those which have been subjected to the moulding or shaping process). Nutrition is an addition to these, without expansion.

VI Let us speak then, in the first place, of genesis, which, as we have said, results from *alteration* together with *shaping*.

The seed having been cast into the womb or into the earth (for there is no difference), then, after a certain definite period, a great number of parts become constituted in the substance which is being generated; these differ as regards moisture, dryness, coldness and warmth, and in all the other qualities which naturally derive therefrom. [. . .]

Now nature constructs bone, cartilage, nerve, membrane, ligament, vein, and so forth, at the first stage of the animal's genesis, employing at this task a faculty which is, in general terms, generative and alterative, and, in more detail, warming, chilling, drying, or moistening; or such as spring from the blending of these, for example the bone-producing, nerve-producing and cartilage-producing faculties (since for the sake of clearness these names must be used as well).

Now the peculiar flesh [parenchyma] of the liver is of this kind as well, also that of the spleen, that of the kidneys, that of the lungs and that of the heart; so also the proper substance of the brain, stomach, gullet, intestines, and uterus is *a sensible element*, of similar parts all through, simple, and uncompounded. That is to say, if you remove from each of the organs mentioned its arteries, veins, and nerves, the substance remaining in each organ is, from the point of view of the senses, simple and elementary. As regards those organs consisting of two dissimilar *coats*, of which each is simple, of these organs the coats are the elements – for example, the coats of the stomach, oesophagus, intestines and arteries; each of these two coats has an alterative faculty peculiar to it, which has engendered it from the menstrual blood of the mother. Thus the *special* alterative faculties in each animal are of the same number as the elementary parts [i.e. tissues]; and further, the *activities* must necessarily correspond each to one of the special parts, just as each part has its special *use* – for example, those ducts which extend from the kidneys into the bladder, and which are called *ureters*; for these are not arteries, since they do not pulsate nor do they consist of two coats; and they are not veins, since they neither contain blood, nor do their coats in any way resemble those of veins; from nerves they differ still more than from the structures mentioned.

'What, then, are they?' someone asks – as though every part must necessarily be either an artery, a vein, a nerve, or a complex of these, and as though the truth were not what I am now stating, namely, that every one of the various organs has its own particular substance. For in fact the two bladders – that which receives the urine, and that which receives the yellow bile – not only differ from all other organs, but also from one another. Further, the ducts which spring out like kinds of conduits from the gall-bladder and which pass into the liver have no resemblance either to arteries, veins or nerves. [. . .]

As for the actual substance of the coats of the stomach, intestine, and uterus, each of these has been rendered what it is by a special alterative faculty of nature; while the bringing of these together, the combination therewith of the structures which are inserted into them, the outgrowth into the intestine, the shape of the inner cavities, and the like, have all been determined by a faculty which we call the shaping or formative faculty; this faculty we also state to be *artistic* – nay, the best and highest art – doing everything for some purpose, so that there is nothing ineffective or superfluous, or capable of being better disposed.

VII Passing now to the faculty of growth let us first mention that this, too, is present in the foetus *in utero* as is also the nutritive faculty, but that at that stage these two faculties are, as it were, *handmaids* to those already mentioned, and do not possess in themselves supreme authority. When, however, the animal has attained its complete size, then, during the whole period following its birth and until the acme is reached, the faculty of growth is predominant, while the alterative and nutritive faculties are accessory – in fact, act as its handmaids. What, then, is the property of this faculty of growth? To extend in every direction that which has already come into existence – that is to say, the solid parts of the body, the arteries, veins, nerves, bones, cartilages, membranes, ligaments, and the various *coats* which we have just called elementary, homogeneous and simple. And I shall state in what way they gain this extension in every direction, first giving an illustration for the sake of clearness.

Children take the bladders of pigs, fill them with air, and then rub them on ashes near the fire, so as to warm, but not to injure them. This is a common game in the district of Ionia, and among not a few other nations. As they rub, they sing songs, to a certain measure, time and rhythm, and all their words are an exhortation to the bladder to increase in size. When it appears to them fairly well distended, they again blow air into it and expand it further; then they rub it again. This they do several times, until the bladder seems to them to have become large enough. Now, clearly, in these doings of the children, the more the interior cavity of the bladder increases in size, the thinner, necessarily, does its substance become. But, if the children were able to bring nourishment to this thin part, then they would make the bladder big in the same way that nature does. As it is, however, they cannot do what nature does, for to imitate this is beyond the power not only of children, but of any one soever; it is a property of nature alone.

It will now, therefore, be clear to you that *nutrition* is a necessity for growing things. For if such bodies were distended, but not at the same time nourished, they would take on a false appearance of growth, not a true growth. And further, to be distended *in all directions* belongs only to bodies whose growth is directed by nature; for those which are distended by us undergo this distension in one direction but grow less in the others; it is impossible to find a body which will remain entire and not be torn through whilst we stretch it in the three dimensions. Thus nature alone has the power to expand a body in all directions so that it remains unruptured and preserves completely its previous form.

Such then is growth, and it cannot occur without the nutriment which flows to the part and is worked up into it.

VIII We have, then, it seems, arrived at the subject of nutrition, which is the third and remaining consideration which we proposed at the outset. For, when the matter which flows to each part of the body in the form of nutriment is being worked up into it, this activity is *nutrition*, and its cause is the *nutritive faculty*. Of course, the kind of activity here involved is also an alteration, but not an alteration like that occurring at the stage of genesis. For in the latter case something comes into existence which did not exist previously, while in nutrition the inflowing material becomes assimilated to that which has already come into existence. Therefore, the former kind of alteration has with reason been termed genesis, and the latter, *assimilation*.

IX [. . .] Genesis, growth, and nutrition are the first, and, so to say, the principal effects of nature; similarly also the faculties which produce these effects – the first faculties – are three in number, and are the most dominating of all. But as has already been shown, these need the service both of each other, and of yet different faculties. Now these which the faculties of generation and growth require have been stated. I shall now say what ones the nutritive faculty requires.

X For I believe that I shall prove that the organs which have to do with the disposal of the nutriment, as also their faculties, exist for the sake of this nutritive faculty. For since the action of this faculty is assimilation, and it is impossible for anything to be assimilated by, and to change into anything else unless they already possess a certain *community and affinity* in their qualities, therefore, in the first place, any animal cannot naturally derive nourishment from any kind of food, and secondly, even in the case of those from which it can do so, it cannot do this at once. Therefore, by reason of this law, every animal needs several organs for *altering* the nutriment. For in order that the yellow may become red, and the red yellow, one simple process of alteration is required, but in order that the white may become black, and the black white, all the intermediate stages are needed. So also, a thing which is very soft cannot all at once become very hard, nor vice versa; nor, similarly can anything which has a very bad smell suddenly become quite fragrant, nor again can the converse happen.

How, then, could blood ever turn into bone, without having first become, as far as possible, thickened and white? And how could bread turn into blood without having gradually parted with its whiteness and gradually acquired redness? Thus it is quite easy for blood to become flesh; for, if nature thicken it to such an extent that it acquires a certain consistency and ceases to be fluid, it thus becomes original newly-formed flesh; but in order that blood may turn into bone, much time is needed and much elaboration and transformation of the blood. Further, it is quite clear that bread, and, more particularly lettuce, beet, and the like, require a great deal of alteration in order to become blood.

This, then, is one reason why there are so many organs concerned in the alteration of food. A second reason is the nature of the *superfluities*. For, as we are unable to draw any nourishment from grass, although this is possible for cattle, similarly we can derive nourishment from radishes, albeit not to the same extent as from meat; for almost the whole of the latter is mastered by our natures; it is transformed and altered and constituted useful blood; but, in the radish, what is appropriate and capable of being altered (and that only with difficulty, and with much labour) is the very smallest part; almost the whole of it is surplus matter, and passes through the digestive organs, only a very little being taken up into the veins as blood. Nature, therefore, had need of a second process of separation for the superfluities in the veins. Moreover, these superfluities need, on the one hand, certain fresh routes to conduct them to the outlets, so that they may not spoil the useful substances, and they also need certain *reservoirs*, as it were, in which they are collected till they reach a sufficient quantity, and are then discharged.

Thus, then, you have discovered bodily parts of a second kind, consecrated in this case to the [removal of the] superfluities of the food. There is, however, also a third kind, for carrying the pabulum in every direction; these are like a number of roads intersecting the whole body.

Thus there is one entrance – that through the mouth – for all the various articles of food. What receives nourishment, however, is not one single part, but a great many parts, and these widely separated; do not be surprised, therefore, at the abundance of organs which nature has created for the purpose of nutrition. For those of them which have to do with alteration prepare the nutriment suitable for each part; others separate out the superfluities; some pass these along, others store them up, others excrete them; some, again, are paths for the transit in all directions of the *utilizable* juices. So, if you wish to gain a thorough acquaintance with all the faculties of nature, you will have to consider each one of these organs.

Now in giving an account of these we must begin with those effects of nature, together with their corresponding parts and faculties, which are closely connected with the purpose to be achieved.

[. . .]

XIII [. . .] For those people who do not believe that there exists in any part of the animal a faculty for attracting *its own special quality* are compelled repeatedly to deny obvious facts. For instance, Asclepiades the physician did this in the case of the kidneys. That these are organs for secreting the urine, was the belief not only of Hippocrates and all other physicians of eminence, but practically every butcher is aware of this, from the fact that he daily observes both the position of the kidneys and the duct (termed the ureter) which runs from each kidney into the bladder, and from this arrangement he infers their characteristic use and faculty. [. . .]

It is worthwhile, then, learning how his theory accounts for the presence of urine in the bladder, and one is forced to marvel at the ingenuity of a man who puts aside these broad, clearly visible routes, [the ureters] and postulates others which are narrow, invisible – indeed, entirely imperceptible. His view, in fact, is that the fluid which we drink passes into the bladder by being resolved into vapours, and that, when these have been again condensed, it thus regains its previous form, and turns from vapour into fluid. He simply looks upon the bladder as a sponge or a piece of wool, and not as the perfectly compact and impervious body that it is, with two very strong coats. For if we say that the vapours pass through these coats, why should they not pass through the peritoneum and the diaphragm, thus filling the whole abdominal cavity and thorax with water? 'But,' says he, 'of course the peritoneal coat is more impervious than the bladder, and this is why it keeps out the vapours, while the bladder admits them.' Yet if he had ever practised anatomy, he might have known that the outer coat of the bladder springs from the peritoneum and is essentially the same as it, and that the inner coat, which is peculiar to the bladder, is more than twice as thick as the former.

Perhaps, however, it is not the thickness or thinness of the coats, but the *situation* of the bladder, which is the reason for the vapours being carried into it? On the contrary, even if it were probable for every other reason that the vapours accumulate there, yet the situation of the bladder would be enough in itself to prevent this. For the bladder is situated below, whereas vapours have a natural tendency to rise upwards; thus they would fill all the region of the thorax and lungs long before they came to the bladder.

[. . .]

The fact is that those who are enslaved to their sects are not merely devoid of all sound knowledge, but they will not even stop to learn! Instead of listening, as they ought, to the reason why liquid can enter the bladder through the ureters, but is unable to go back again the same way, – instead of admiring nature's artistic skill – they refuse to learn; they even go so far as to scoff, and maintain that the kidneys, as well as many other things, have been made by nature *for no purpose*! And some of them who had allowed themselves to be shown the ureters coming from the kidneys and becoming implanted in the bladder, even had the audacity to say that these also existed for no purpose; and others said that they were spermatic ducts, and that this was why they were inserted into the neck of the bladder and not into its cavity. [. . .] We were, therefore, further compelled to show them in a still living animal, the urine plainly running out through the ureters into the bladder; even thus we hardly hoped to check their nonsensical talk.

Now the method of demonstration is as follows. One has to divide the peritoneum in front of the ureters, then secure these with ligatures, and next, having bandaged up the animal, let him go (for he will not continue to urinate). After this one loosens the external bandages and shows the bladder empty and the ureters quite full and distended – in fact almost on the point of rupturing; on removing the ligature from them, one then plainly sees the bladder becoming filled with urine.

When this has been made quite clear, then, before the animal urinates, one has to tie a ligature round his penis and then to squeeze the bladder all over; still nothing goes back through the ureters to the kidneys. Here, then, it becomes obvious that not only in a dead animal, but in one which is still living, the ureters are prevented from receiving back the urine from the bladder. These observations having been made, one now loosens the ligature from the animal's penis and allows him to urinate, then again ligatures one of the ureters and leaves the other to discharge into the bladder. Allowing some time to elapse, one now demonstrates that the ureter which was ligatured is obviously full and distended on the side next to the kidneys, while the other one – that from which the ligature had been taken – is itself flaccid, but has filled the bladder with urine. Then, again, one must divide the full ureter, and demonstrate how the urine spurts out of it, like blood in the operation of venesection; and after this one cuts through the other also, and both being thus divided, one bandages up the animal externally. Then when enough time seems to have elapsed, one takes off the bandages; the bladder will now be found empty, and the whole region between the intestines and the peritoneum full of urine, as if the animal were suffering from dropsy. Now, if anyone will but test this for himself on an animal, I think he will strongly condemn the rashness of Asclepiades, and if he also learns the reason why nothing regurgitates from the bladder into the ureters, I think he will be persuaded by this also of the forethought and art shown by nature in relation to animals.

[. . .]

XV [. . .] Most assuredly, either the urine is conveyed by its own motion to the kidneys, considering this the better course [. . .], or, if this be impossible, then some other reason for its conveyance must be found. What, then, is this? If we are not going to grant the kidneys a faculty for attracting this particular quality, as Hippocrates held, we shall discover no other reason. For, surely everyone sees that either the kidneys must attract the urine, or the veins must propel it – if, that is, it does not move of itself. But if the veins did exert a propulsive action when they contract, they would squeeze out into the kidneys not merely the urine, but along with it the whole of the blood which they contain. And if this is impossible, as we shall show, the remaining explanation is that the kidneys do exert traction.

And how is propulsion by the veins impossible? The situation of the kidneys is against it. They do not occupy a position beneath the hollow vein [vena cava] as does the sieve-like [ethmoid] passage in the nose and palate in relation to the surplus matter from the brain; they are situated on both sides of it. Besides, if the kidneys are like sieves, and readily let the thinner serous [whey-like] portion through and keep out the thicker portion, then the whole of the blood contained in the vena cava must go to them, just as the whole of the wine is thrown into the filters. Further, the example of milk being made into cheese will show clearly what I mean. For this, too, although it is all thrown into the wicker strainers, does not all percolate through; such part of it as is too fine in proportion to the width of the meshes passes downwards, and this is called *whey* [serum]; the remaining thick portion which is destined to become cheese cannot get down, since the pores of the strainers will not admit it. Thus it is that if the blood-serum has similarly to percolate through the kidneys, the whole of the blood must come to them, and not merely one part of it.

What, then, is the appearance as found on dissection?

One division of the vena cava is carried upwards to the heart, and the other mounts upon the spine and extends along its whole length as far as the legs; thus one division does not even come near the kidneys, while the other approaches them but is certainly not inserted into them. Now, if the blood were destined to be purified by them as if they were sieves, the whole of it would have to fall into them, the thin part being thereafter conveyed downwards, and the thick part retained above. But, as a matter of fact, this is not so. For the kidneys lie on either side of the vena cava. They therefore do not act like sieves, filtering fluid sent to them by the vena cava, and themselves contributing no force. They obviously exert traction; for this is the only remaining alternative.

[. . .]

XVI [. . .] In relation to the lower part of the vena cava there would still remain, solitary and abandoned, the specious theory concerning the filling of a vacuum. This, however, is deprived of plausibility by the fact that people die of retention of urine, and also, no less, by the situation of the kidneys. For, if the whole of the blood were carried to the kidneys, one might properly maintain that it all undergoes purification there. But, as a matter of fact, the whole of it does not go to them, but only so much as can be contained in the veins going to the kidneys; this portion only, therefore, will be purified. Further, the thin serous part of this will pass through the kidneys as if through a sieve, while the thick sanguineous portion remaining in the veins will obstruct the blood flowing in from behind; this will first, therefore, have to run back to the vena cava, and so to empty the veins going to the kidneys; these veins will no longer be able to conduct a second quantity of unpurified blood to the kidneys, occupied as they are by the blood which had preceded, there is no passage left. What power have we, then, which will draw back the purified blood from the kidneys? And what power, in the next place, will bid this blood retire to the lower part of the vena cava, and will enjoin on another quantity coming from above not to proceed downwards before turning off into the kidneys?

Now Erasistratus realized that all these ideas were open to many objections, and he could only find one idea which held good in all respects – namely, that of *attraction*. Since, therefore, he did not wish either to get into difficulties or to mention the view of Hippocrates, he deemed it better to say nothing at all as to the manner in which secretion occurs.

But even if he kept silence, I am not going to do so. For I know that if one passes over the Hippocratic view and makes some other pronouncement about the function of the kidneys, one cannot fail to make oneself utterly ridiculous. It was for this reason that Erasistratus kept silence and Asclepiades lied; they are like slaves who have had plenty to say in the early part of their career, and have managed by excessive rascality to escape many and frequent accusations, but who, later, when caught in the act of thieving, cannot find any excuse; the more modest one then keeps silence, as though thunderstruck, whilst the more shameless continues to hide the missing article beneath his arm and denies on oath that he has ever seen it. For it was in this way also that Asclepiades, when all subtle excuses had failed him and there was no longer any room for nonsense about 'conveyance towards the rarefied part [of the air]', and when it was impossible without incurring the greatest derision to say that this super-fluity [i.e. the urine] is generated by the kidneys as is bile by the canals in the liver – he then, I say, clearly lied when he swore that the urine does not reach the kidneys, and maintained that it passes, in the form of vapour, straight from the region of the vena cava, to collect in the bladder.

Like slaves, then, caught in the act of stealing, these two are quite bewildered, and while the one says nothing, the other indulges in shameless lying.

XVII [. . .] Now those near the times of Erasistratus maintain that the parts above the kidneys receive pure blood, whilst the watery residue, being heavy, tends to run downwards; that this, after percolating through the kidneys themselves, is thus rendered serviceable, and is sent, as blood, to all the parts below the kidneys.

For a certain period at least this view also found favour and flourished, and was held to be true; after a time, however, it became suspect to the Erasistrateans themselves, and at last they abandoned it. For apparently, the following two points were assumed, neither of which is conceded by anyone, nor is even capable of being proved. The first is the heaviness of the serous fluid, which was said to be produced in the vena cava, and which did not exist, apparently, at the beginning, when this fluid was being carried up from the stomach to the liver. Why, then, did it not at once run downwards when it was in these situations ?[. . .]

In the second place there is this absurdity, that even if it be agreed that all the watery fluid does fall downwards, and only when it is in the vena cava, still it is difficult, or, rather, impossible, to say through what means it is going to fall into the kidneys, seeing that these are not situated below, but on either side of the vena cava, and that the vena cava is not inserted into them, but merely sends a branch into each of them, as it also does into all the other parts.

[. . .] I dwell purposely on this topic, knowing well that nobody else has anything to say about the function of the kidneys, but that either we must prove more foolish than the very butchers if we do not agree that the urine passes through the kidneys; or, if one acknowledges this, that then one cannot possibly give any other reason for the secretion than the principle of attraction.

Part Two **Revolt**

Andreas Vesalius

Vesalius was one of the major figures in redirecting the current of medical thought. Born in 1514, he had his preliminary education at Louvain, studied at the University of Paris and finally went to Padua, where he received his medical degree in 1537. Immediately he became professor of anatomy at this famous university. His greatest work, the *De humanis corporis fabrica*, renowned for its superb illustrations, he published in 1543. From our standpoint the significance of Vesalius lies in his empirical methodology. He wanted to see for himself and he refused to accept the authority of Galen in matters of fact. He insisted on performing his own dissections, and thereby departed from the earlier tradition wherein a professor teaching anatomy read from a book, while a person of much lower status performed the actual prosection.

We must not think that Vesalius at a single stroke brought medicine from a tradition-bound and authoritative past to a scientific present. He often accepted unscientifically what earlier writers had said, and he himself made numerous errors of observation. Nevertheless he took a great step forward in the development of medicine as an observational science. He emphasized new attitudes and new standards.

Vesalius dedicated his book to Charles V and our selection comes from the Preface. In it Vesalius indicated the relatively low state of contemporary medicine, so far as its actual practice was concerned. In the great days of classical medicine, the physician was not only a theorist but also a therapeutist, who worked with his hands as well as with his mind. During medieval development, the practitioners of medicine were learned men of great education who devoted themselves more and more to affairs of the mind rather than of the hands. Practical manual activity, whether it involved dissection or surgery or practical therapeutics, was beneath the dignity of the physician, and was relegated to the lower classes of practitioners.

During the medieval period medicine had become progressively more remote from reality and correspondingly more speculative – concerned with rational elaboration and logical inference rather than with observation. Vesalius tried to reverse the trend, and he emphasized the importance of seeing and doing, rather than merely speculating or performing logical gymnastics.

The excerpts from the Preface given here reveal the practical and empirical aspects of medical science in the early Renaissance. In the sixteenth century there was very little scope for exactness in science, and anatomy represented the only branch of medicine where precision could have full sway. Actually, greater precision in the field of anatomy, and more accurate descriptions of nature, really had very little practical effect on the practice of medicine. The surgery of the day was quite crude, and a more precise knowledge of fine points of anatomy did not find any reflection in better or more effective surgery. The interest in precise description influenced much more the attitude of physicians than the practical treatment of patients. And it is this changed attitude which is supremely important in understanding the transformation of medicine during the past five hundred years.

4 De Humanis Corporis Fabrica (1543)

Excerpts from 'The Preface of Andreas Vesalius to his Books *De humanis corporis fabrica*', in C. D. O'Malley, *Andreas Vesalius of Brussels 1514–1564*, University of California Press, 1964, pp. 317–23.

[. . .] Once there were three medical sects – Dogmatic, Empirical, and Methodical – but their members consulted the whole art as the means of preserving health and driving away sicknesses. All the thoughts of each sect were directed toward this goal and three methods were employed: The first was a regimen of diet, the second the use of drugs, and the third the use of the hands.[. . .] This triple method of treatment was equally familiar to the physicians of each sect, and those using their own hands according to the nature of the sickness used no less effort in training them than in establishing a theory of diet or in understanding and compounding drugs.

[. . .]

Especially after the devastation of the Goths, when all the sciences, formerly so flourishing and fittingly practised, had decayed, the more fashionable physicians, first in Italy in imitation of the old Romans, despising the use of the hands, began to relegate to their slaves those things which had to be done manually for their patients and to stand over them like architects. Then when, by degrees, others who practised true medicine also declined those unpleasant duties – not, however, reducing their fees or dignity – they promptly degenerated from the earlier physicians, leaving the method of cooking and all the preparation of the patients' diet to nurses, the composition of drugs to apothecaries, and the use of the hands to barbers. And so in the course of time the art of treatment has been so miserably distorted that certain doctors assuming the name of physicians have arrogated to themselves the prescription of drugs and diet for obscure diseases, and have relegated the rest of medicine to those whom they call surgeons, but consider scarcely as slaves. They have shamefully rid themselves of what is the chief and most venerable branch of medicine, that which based itself principally upon the investigation of nature. [. . .]

I certainly do not propose to give preference to one instrument of medicine over the others, since the aforesaid triple method of treatment can in no way be disunited and the whole of it belongs to the one practitioner; and that he may employ it properly all parts of medicine have been equally established so that the successful use of a single part depends upon the degree to which they are all combined, for how rare is the sickness that does not immediately require the three instruments of treatment. Hence a proper scheme of diet must be determined, and something must be done with drugs, and finally with the hands, so that the tyros of this art ought – if it please the gods – to be urged in every way, like the Greeks, to scorn the whisperings of those physicians and, as nature teaches, to employ their hands in treatment, lest they convert the mangled rationale of treatment into a calamity for the life of mankind. They ought to be urged the more strongly to this since we see learned physicians abstain from the use of the hands as from a plague lest the rabbins of medicine decry them before the ignorant mass as barbers and they acquire less wealth and honour than those [who are] scarcely half-physicians, and stand in less estimation before the uncomprehending mass of the people. Indeed, it is especially this detestable, vulgar opinion that prevents us, even in our age, from taking up the art of treatment as a whole, limiting us to the treatment of only internal diseases, to the great harm of mankind, and – if I may speak frankly – we strive to be physicians only in part.

When first the whole composition of drugs was relegated to the apothecaries, then the physicians promptly lost the necessary knowledge of simple medicines, and they were responsible for the apothecaries' shops becoming filled with barbarous names, and even false remedies, and for so many admirable compositions of the ancients being lost to us, several of which are still missing.

[. . .]

For when the physicians assumed that only the treatment of internal complaints concerned them, believing furthermore that knowledge of only the viscera was sufficient, they neglected the structure of the bones, muscles and nerves, and of the veins and arteries which creep through those bones and muscles, as of no concern to them. In addition, when the use of the hands was wholly entrusted to the barbers, not only was true knowledge of the viscera lost to the physicians, but also the practice of dissection soon died away, because they did not undertake it, and those to whom the manual skills had been entrusted were so unlearned that they did not understand the writings of the professors of dissection.

Thus it was impossible that so very difficult and abstruse an art, acquired mechanically by this latter type of men, could be preserved for us, for the deplorable division of the art of treatment introduced into the schools that detestable procedure by which usually some conduct the dissection of the human body and others present the account of its parts, the latter like jackdaws aloft in their high chair, with egregious arrogance croaking things they have never investigated but merely committed to memory from the books of others, or reading what has already been described. The former are so ignorant of languages that they are unable to explain their dissections to the spectators and muddle what ought to be displayed according to the instructions of the physician who, since he has never applied his hand to the dissection of the body, haughtily governs the ship from a manual. Thus everything is wrongly taught in the schools, and days are wasted in ridiculous questions so that in such confusion less is presented to the spectators than a butcher in his stall could teach a physician. [. . .]

They [the contemporary anatomists] are so firmly dependent upon I-know-not-what-quality in the writing of their leader that, coupled with the failure of others to dissect, they have shamefully reduced Galen into brief compendia and never depart from him – if ever they understood his meaning – by the breadth of a nail. Indeed, in the prefaces of their books they announce that their writings are wholly pieced together from Galen's conclusions and that all that is theirs is his, adding that if anyone by chance were to criticize their writings they would consider that Galen also had been criticized. So completely have all yielded to him that there is no physician who would declare that even the slightest error had ever been found, much less can now be found, in Galen's anatomical books, although – except that Galen often corrects himself, frequently alluding to his negligence in earlier books and often teaching the opposite in later ones after he became more experienced – it is now clear to me from the reborn art of dissection, from diligent reading of Galen's books and their restoration in several places – for which we need feel no shame – that he never dissected a human body; but deceived by his monkeys – although he did have access to two dried human cadavers – he frequently and improperly opposed the ancient physicians trained in human dissection. Nay, more, how many incorrect observations you will find in Galen, even regarding his monkeys, not to mention that it is very astonishing that Galen noticed none of the many and infinite differences between the organs of the human body and of the monkey except in the fingers and the bend of the knee, which undoubtedly he would have overlooked with the others except that they were obvious to him without human dissection.

However, at present I do not intend to criticize the false teachings of Galen, easily prince of professors of dissection; much less do I wish to be considered as disloyal from the start to the author of all good things and as paying no heed to his authority. For I recollect how the physicians – far otherwise than the followers of Aristotle – are usually upset when in the conduct of a single anatomy nowadays they see Galen's description to have been incorrect in well over two hundred instances relating to the human structure and its use and function, and how examining the dissected parts they seek fiercely and with the greatest zeal to defend him. Nevertheless, even they, influenced by love of truth, have little by little subsided and put more faith into their not-ineffectual eyes and reason than in Galen's writings. [. . .]

I have done my best to this single end, to aid as many as possible in a very recondite as well as laborious matter, and truly and completely to describe the structure of the human body which is formed not of ten or twelve parts – as it may seem to the spectator – but of some thousands of different parts, and, among other monuments to that divine man Galen, to bring to posterity an understanding of those books of his requiring the help of a teacher. I bear to the candidates of medicine fruit not to be scorned.

I am aware that by reason of my age – I am at present twenty-eight years old – my efforts will have little authority, and that, because of my frequent indication of the falsity of Galen's teachings, they will find little shelter from the attacks of those who were not present at my anatomical demonstrations or have not themselves studied the subject sedulously; various schemes in defence of Galen will be boldly invented unless these books appear with the auspicious commendation and great patronage of some divine power. Because they cannot be more safely sheltered or more splendidly adorned than by the imperishable name of the great and invincible emperor, the divine Charles, I beseech your imperial Majesty with all reverence again and again, to permit this youthful work of mine to come into the hands of men – to whom for many reasons it is obnoxious – for a short time, under your splendid patronage, until through the experience, judgement and erudition that come with age I may render it more worthy of so great a prince or I may offer another acceptable gift on some other subject taken from our art.

Padua, 1 August 1542

Paracelsus

The Renaissance had two quite distinct trends. One, grounded in philosophy and metaphysics, was essentially speculative with a small basis in fact and a large superstructure of theory. An opposing trend promoted observation and the recording of facts, and discouraged speculations. Vesalius, empirically oriented, had an intense concern for facts. Paracelsus, in marked contrast, was devoted to theoretical, speculative and philosophic considerations.

Paracelsus (1493–1541), whose real name was Hohenheim, was born in Switzerland. He apparently had some personality defects, as indicated by his incessant wanderings and inability to adapt for any length of time in any one place. His constant rebellion against authority and his continuously antagonistic manner bear out this defect. He is difficult to understand, and critics have been more apt to revile him than to examine his views sympathetically. Only in this century has he begun to be appreciated, under the influence of such writers as Sudhoff and Pagel.

To understand Paracelsus we must realize that he shared in the neoplatonic tradition, that is, in the belief in a continuity of existence – of Being – beginning with the immaterial divine One. Through a series of gradations this spiritual existence became progressively more 'dilute'. In its progressive gradations, the divine existence became transformed, and gave rise to mind, soul and various heavenly creatures – the stars, the Earth, its inhabitants and eventually its material substance. The teachings of Paracelsus are in this neoplatonic tradition, although by no means merely a copy.

We must emphasize that Paracelsus was not searching for facts, as was Vesalius. He had an insight into the nature of the universe, and the interrelations of various components, and he merely stated his insights, without attempting to prove them. At most he gave certain analogies which do not have any logical cogency, any more than does the insight of a poet.

The present quotations come from one of his important writings dealing with the various bases to which disease can be attributed. He called these *entia* – existences – by which he meant the basic categories of being that are relevant to health. Paracelsus realized that vast forces of extreme complexity were at work in the universe, and that there were interrelations between different components. His conception of the *mysterium magnum* is that of an all-pervading matrix in which we live and have our being, a sort of metaphysical atmosphere which makes possible various interactions. The *mysterium magnum* affects our health in various ways. Paracelsus thought that many of the relevant influences derived from the stars, which represented, so to speak, a stage in the transmission of divine influence.

One category that concerns disease he characterized by the term poison. In his discussion he indicated some aspects of what we would call metabolism, and the way one living creature, with a characteristic metabolism, differs sharply from another. When he indicated that certain bodily functions were under the control of an alchemist, he meant that the bodily processes are essentially chemical in nature, having a kinship with the chemical processes outside the body. He believed that the internal chemistry of one animal species is very different from that of another. Metabolic process natural to one species is quite foreign to a different species, and not only foreign but 'poisonous'.

In these selections we can give only the barest hint of the doctrines of Paracelsus. He had a vast influence on subsequent thought, particularly in the seventeenth century, and is worthy of more detailed study.

5 Volumen Medicinae Paramirum (?1529)

Excerpts from Paracelsus (Theophrastus von Hohenheim), 'Volumen medicinae Paramirum', translated by Kurt F. Leidecker, in Owsei Temkin (ed.), *Supplements to the Bulletin of the History of Medicine*, Johns Hopkins Press, 1949, pp. 18–33.

Tract concerning the 'Ens Astrale'

Chapter the sixth

[. . .] You should understand by *Ens Astrale* the following. It is something we do not see, something which sustains life in us and in everything that is alive and sentient. This something derives from the heavenly bodies. To illustrate: a fire which burns must have wood, otherwise there would be no fire. Thus you observe that fire is a vital thing, yet it cannot live without wood. Now for the application. Although this is too clumsy an illustration you must bear with it. The body is the wood, the life within it the fire. Now, life derives its substance from the body. Consequently, the body must possess something which prevents it from being consumed by life but, on the contrary, continues to exist. That is the thing concerning which we tell you as the *Ens*. It hails from the firmament. You say, and rightly so, if there were no air, all things would fall to the ground, and all that has life here below would stifle and die. By the same token remember that there is something else that sustains the body, the same body which sustains life. That you may do without as little as the air. The air is sustained in and by this something; this away, and the air would disappear. The firmament lives by virtue of this something, and if it were not in the firmament, the firmament would vanish. That something we call the M[YSTERIUM]. For there is nothing in the whole universe created above this, nothing higher, nothing is more important for the physician to bear in mind. Observe now carefully: this M[YSTERIUM], we say, does not originate in the firmament, nor has it sprung from it, nor does the firmament send it to us – nothing of the kind. Nevertheless mark well that this M[YSTERIUM] is supporting all creatures, in heaven and on earth; and all elements live by and in it. [. . .]

Chapter the seventh

Take, first of all, a simile in explanation of the M[YSTERIUM]. A chamber, in which the air has been befouled by you and whose doors are shut, receives the odour that you have imparted it. This odour does not come from the chamber, it comes from you. Now take note: just as you create this odour, so must those scent it who are in it; and it is possible that for all those dwelling in the chamber you may be responsible for all their diseases as well as cures. That is to say, the air which is in the chamber does not come from you, but the odour comes from you.

[. . .] The M[YSTERIUM] M[AGNUM] is such that all creatures live by it and have their lives in and through it. This M[YSTERIUM] M[AGNUM] may be poisoned and changed and man may thus be obliged to take it up into himself. As long as his life is and dwells within the M[YSTERIUM] M[AGNUM], so long does his body have no choice, but must suffer to have what is in the M[YSTERIUM] M[AGNUM] poured out over him, and be polluted by it – just as in the case above cited where the air that was in the chamber had been converted. In like manner there may be something that pollutes this M[YSTERIUM], it might stay with it but does not originate from it.

Chapter the eighth

Thus, the *Ens Astrorum* is to be understood as follows: the stars have their nature and their various characteristics just like people on earth. These same stars undergo changes within, be it for better or for worse, for sweeter or sourer, for greater pungency or bitterness. Thus, if they are well disposed, nothing evil emanates from them; but when they are evil disposed, their wickedness comes to the fore. Now, you should know that they surround the entire world like the shell of an egg. Air penetrates through the shell and first passes through it toward the center of the world. Stars, mind you, which are poisonous, pollute the air with their poison. Accordingly, wherever the poison penetrates, on that same spot the identical diseases will crop out in conformity to the character of the star in question. To be sure, the entire air in the world is not poisoned by the star, but merely a part thereof, depending on its strength. It is likewise so with the good qualities of the stars.

Ens Astrale thus signifies the odour, vapour, exudation of the stars as mixed with air, as is demonstrated by *Cursus Astrorum* (the course of the stars). It is in this manner that we get cold, heat, dryness, moisture and the like, as indicated by their properties. It is well to bear thus in mind that the heavenly bodies do not cause propensities in anything. However, through their vapours, they pollute the M[YSTERIUM], by which we in turn are being polluted and weakened. Of such a nature is, thus, the *Ens Astrale* that it influences the body in such a manner for good or ill. Any person who is thus by his very nature antagonistic to a particular vapour, falls sick. But he whose nature is not incompatible with it, derives no harm from it. He also does not suffer harm who is so pure and well fortified against it that he overcomes the poison by virtue of the refined nature of his blood or the medical preparation which resists the corrupted vapours of those beings above. [. . .]

Chapter the ninth

As to the topic M[YSTERIUM], an example may be given to illustrate how the vapours of the planets cause damage to us. A pond, in the possession of its proper M[YSTERIUM], abounds in fishes. If the cold, however, becomes too severe, the pond freezes over and the fishes die because the M[YSTERIUM] is too frigid for the nature of the water. This frigidity does not originate with the M[YSTERIUM], but from the heavenly body which possesses this property and causes same. In the same way acts also the heat of the sun, so that the water becomes too warm and the fishes die for the reasons aforementioned. Just as these two, heat and cold, are two properties of some heavenly bodies bringing such things to pass, so there are others which make the M[YSTERIUM] sour, bitter, sweet, sharp, arsenic and the like to suit many hundred tastes and so forth. This great change of the M[YSTERIUM] is equivalent to changes in the body. Be on the lookout for the way in which the heavenly bodies pollute the M[YSTERIUM] causing us to fall sick and die, depending on the nature of their vapours. No physician should be surprised at that. For, however many kinds of poison there are on earth, there are as many and more in the stars. Let each physician be reminded that no disease is produced without a poison. For poison is the origin of every disease, and all diseases are brought on by poison, be they of the body or a wound, nothing excluded. [. . .]

Tract concerning the 'Ens Veneni'

Chapter the first

[. . .]

You know that man's body must have a sustenance, that is a driving force by which it is kept up and nourished; and where that is lacking, there is no life. Therefore, take to heart that he who created and made our body, made the food as well as the body, but not so perfect. Understand this to mean that the body has been given us without poison, and there is no poison in it. But in what we must offer the body as food, in that there is poison. In other words, the body has been created perfect, but not the other. Now, in that other animals and fruit are food for us, they may also be poison to us. However, as far as they themselves are concerned, they are neither poison nor food. In themselves they are creatures as perfect as we are. Yet, when they become food for us, they constitute a poison for us. What is not poison for itself is nevertheless poison for us.

Chapter the second

[. . .]

[God] has appointed an alchemist for us to convert the imperfect which we have to utilize into something useful to us so that we may not consume the poison which we take in amongst the things that are good, as a poison, but eliminate it from the good.
[. . .]

Chapter the third

Since every thing, in itself, is perfect but in relation to some other thing is either a poison or a good, our reasoning leads us to believe that God has appointed an alchemist for him who has to use the other for an end and which enters him, or is administered to him, as a poison or something beneficent. Such a great artist is he that he segregates the two, the poison in its proper bag, the good substance into the body. In the manner indicated it behooves you to understand and recognize well our thesis.
[. . .]

Chapter the fourth

Understand the Creator thus: All things are perfect in themselves, and it has been decreed by the Creator that one must sustain the other, grass the cow, the cow man. Thus, the perfection of one thing being good and evil and imperfect with respect to another which consumes it, has caused Him to create something else. [. . .] He has brought it about that in the thing which another being must utilize, there is a quality, an ability and dexterity such that by virtue of it the poison is sifted from the good at no injury to body and food. This is how it operates.

Take as an example the following. The peacock eats snakes, lizards and stellions; these are animals that are perfect in themselves and healthy, yet when required by other animals they are rank poison, except to the peacock. But as to the reason for this, you should know that the peacock's alchemist is so subtle in thus segregating the poison from the good in things which do not injure the peacock, that no animal is its equal as far as their alchemist is concerned. Remember further that each animal has its own food which is meant to be food especially adapted to it and possesses an alchemist specially assigned it, for doing the segregating.

[. . .]

To the pig, excrements are proper. Although these are a poison (being eliminated for this reason by nature's alchemist from man) they nevertheless serve the pig as food, because the pig's alchemist is yet more subtle than man's alchemist, in that the pig's alchemist extracts food even from the excrements, which man's alchemist has not been able to do. Hence the excrements of the pig are not eaten by any animal whatsoever. For, there is no shrewder alchemist that will analyse food more minutely than the pig's alchemist.

[. . .]

Chapter the thirteenth

[. . .] The oxen, by his constitution, is so created as to satisfy his own need and serve as food for man's nourishment. Now mark that as far as man is concerned, the oxen is poison. Had he been created merely on man's account and not also for his own sake, he would need neither horns, bones nor hoofs. For these do not constitute food, and what becomes of them is nothing that is essential. Accordingly you will observe that he has been created fully adequate to himself and there is nothing on him he could dispense with or would no longer want. But, as soon as man enjoys him as a food, man has to eat also what is contrary to his own nature and constitutes a poison, which, to the oxen, was never poisonous at all. This poison must be eliminated by man's own nature, that is, his alchemist.

William Harvey

While we cannot sharply circumscribe a 'modern' era in medical history we can point to one event that made a sharp break from the past and redirected the whole course of medicine into different channels. That event was Harvey's discovery of the circulation of the blood. When Harvey, in 1628, demonstrated that the blood moved in a circle, he changed the orientation of medical thought. The change came about gradually but inexorably.

Harvey was born in 1578, received a good education, matriculated at Cambridge, studied medicine in Padua – receiving his degree in 1602 – and then returned to England. There he built up a successful medical practice, rose rapidly in his professional associations and became court physician in 1618. He enjoyed, as well, a personal friendship with Charles I, and embraced the Royalist cause in the civil war. While Harvey is best known for his studies on the circulation – the famous *De Motu Cordis*, published in 1628 – he also was a capable experimental embryologist, and his *De Generatione Animalium*, published in 1651, has only recently been receiving the attention it deserves.

Harvey's work on the circulation may be considered to have a twofold significance. First there was the factual aspect: the actual discovery. He showed that the heart was a pump which impelled the blood in a continuous fashion into two distinct but connected circuits. The right ventricle pushed the blood into the lungs. After completion of the 'pulmonary transit' the blood entered the left side of the heart. From here, propelled by the pumping action of the heart, it travelled through the aorta and the smaller arteries to the veins. The veins carried the blood back to the right side of the heart, to begin the circuit once again.

This schema of circulation contrasted with the Galenic view that envisioned an ebb and flow, rather than a circular movement, and hypothesized that blood passed from the right side of the heart to the left through invisible pores in the septum, rather than through the lungs.

And yet, the concept that the blood moved in a circle was only a part of Harvey's great contribution to medicine. Other investigators had, in one or another fashion, suggested some sort of circulation. The idea of a pulmonary transit was by no means new. Ibn an Nafis in the thirteenth century, and Servetus and Columbus in the sixteenth, had indicated that the blood passed through the lungs, not through the interventricular septum. In the sixteenth century Leonardo da Vinci and, especially, Andreas Cesalpino, held to some sort of a systemic circulation. But Harvey's great contribution was, in a sense, methodological: he *proved* the existence of a circulation, not merely asserted it or speculated about it. He marshalled his evidence carefully, drew cautious and justifiable inferences, and built up a case that was empirically based and logically sound. His methodology had much in common with the best scholastic argumentation, but was an extension thereof that rested firmly on precise observation, well-defined experiments and brilliant reasoning.

The excerpts here give us a fair idea of his critical methodology and his analytic approach.

6 Movement of the Heart and Blood in Animals (1628)

Excerpts from William Harvey, *Movement of the Heart and Blood in Animals*, translated by Kenneth J. Franklin, Charles C. Thomas (Illinois), and Blackwell Scientific Publications, 1957, pp. 39–87.

The movement and functional activity of the heart

From these and suchlike observations I believe that the movement of the heart will be found to occur as follows.

First the auricle contracts and in so doing sends its content of blood (of which it has abundance as head of the veins, and as the blood store and reservoir) into the ventricle of the heart. When the ventricle is full, the heart raises itself, forthwith tenses all its fibres, contracts the ventricles, and gives a beat. By this means it ejects at once into the arteries the blood discharged into it by the auricle, the right ventricle doing so into the lungs through the vessel which is called the artery-like vein but is, in fact, in both structure and function and in all else an artery, the left ventricle doing so into the aorta and through the arteries to the whole of the body.

Those two movements, one of the auricles and the other of the ventricles, occur successively but so harmoniously and rhythmically that both [appear to] happen together and only one movement can be seen, especially in warmer animals in rapid movement. This is comparable with what happens in machines in which, with one wheel moving another, all seem to be moving at once. It also recalls that mechanical device fitted to firearms in which, on pressure to a trigger, a flint falls and strikes and advances the steel, a spark is evoked and falls upon the powder, the powder is fired and the flame leaps inside and spreads and the ball flies out and enters the target; all these movements, because of their rapidity, seeming to happen at once as in the wink of an eye. In swallowing too it is similar. The root of the tongue is raised and the mouth compressed and the food or drink is driven into the fauces, the larynx is closed by its muscles and by the epiglottis, the top of the gullet is raised and opened by its muscles just as a sack is raised for filling and opened out for receiving, and the food or drink taken in is pressed down by the transverse muscles and pulled down by the longer ones. Nevertheless, all those movements, made by diverse and opposite organs in harmonious and orderly fashion, appear, while they are occurring, to effect one movement and to play one role which we style 'swallowing'.

It obviously happens thus in the moving role played by the heart, which is a sort of swallowing and a transmission of blood from the veins into the arteries. If anyone (with these things in mind) inspects the heart's movement carefully in a vivisection, he will not only see, as I have said, the heart rise up and combine with its auricles in one continuous movement, but he will also note a certain undulation and obscure lateral inclination along the line of the right ventricle, which twists lightly as it carries out this task. When a horse drinks and swallows water, one can see that the swallowing and passage onwards of the water into the stomach occur with successive gullet movements, each one causing a sound and an audible and tangible thrill. In similar fashion, with each of those heart movements there is a transmission of a portion of blood from the veins into the arteries, and during it the occurrence of a pulse which is audible within the chest.

The movement of the heart is thus entirely of this description, and the heart's one role is the transmission of the blood and its propulsion, by means of the arteries, to the extremities everywhere. Hence the pulse which we feel in the arteries is nothing but the inthrust of blood into them from the heart.

We must hereafter inquire and deduce from other observations whether the heart, beyond transferring the blood, giving it local movement and distributing it, adds anything else (warmth, spirit, or finish) to it. For the moment let it suffice to have shown adequately that during the heart-beat, blood is transmitted and conducted from the veins through the cardiac ventricles into the arteries, and distributed to the whole of the body.

This is in some measure conceded by all and is inferred by them from the heart's structure, and from the mechanical arrangement, site, and action of the valves. But they seem to be groping about in the dark and to have errors of vision, and they put together things which are diverse, discrepant and incoherent, and – as shown earlier – base very many of their statements on guesswork.

The greatest cause of indecision and error in this matter seems to me to have been a single one, namely, the close connection of the heart and the lungs in the human subject. When investigators had seen the artery-like vein, and similarly the vein-like artery, disappear in the lungs, they were very much at a loss to see whence or how the right ventricle distributed blood to the body or the left ventricle drew blood from the vena cava. [. . .]

The ways by which the blood is carried from the vena cava into the arteries, or from the right ventricle of the heart into the left one

Since it is probable that the connection of the heart with the lung in man provided, as I have said, the opportunity for going astray, those persons do wrong who while wishing, as all anatomists commonly do, to describe, demonstrate and study the parts of animals, content themselves with looking inside one animal only, namely, man – and that one dead. In this way they merely attempt a universal syllogism on the basis of a particular proposition (like those who think they can construct a science of politics after exploration of a single form of government, or have a knowledge of agriculture through investigation of the character of a single field).

Were they as experienced in the dissection of [living] animals as they are practised in the anatomy of the dead human subject, this matter which keeps all involved in uncertainty would, in my view, be simply and readily clarified.

First, then, in fishes, which as lungless animals have but one ventricle of the heart, the matter is sufficiently proved by direct evidence. For by mere inspection or by inspection after division of the artery (the blood gushing out of it with each heart-beat), it can be openly and visibly demonstrated (as is generally admitted) that the sac of blood lying at the base of the heart and obviously analogous to an auricle, sends blood into the heart, which thereupon clearly passes it on through a pipe or artery or a structure analogous to an artery.

Next, the same can readily be seen in all animals in which there is just one, or for practical purposes one, ventricle as, for example, in the toad, frog, serpents and lizards. In these, though they are reputed to be endowed with lungs in some way inasmuch as they are vocal (I have very many observations on the wonderful arrangement of their lungs and other things of that sort but they are irrelevant here), it is nevertheless clear from direct observation that the blood is carried in the same manner from the veins to the arteries by the beat of the heart. The way is patent, revealed, manifest; there is no difficulty in discerning it, no room for uncertainty about it. For in these animals the position is just as it would be in man had the septum of his heart been perforated or removed, or its two ventricles made into one. In that case, I believe, no one would have had any doubt about the way by which the blood had been able to cross from the veins into the arteries.

As in fact the number of animals without lungs exceeds the number of those with them, and as similarly the number of animals with only one ventricle of the heart exceeds the number of those with two ventricles, it is easy to decide that in the majority of animals, for the most part and on the whole, the blood is transmitted by an obvious route from the veins to the arteries through the chamber of the heart.

It has, moreover, been borne in on me that the same very obviously holds good in the embryos of animals that have lungs. In the foetus, as is well known to anatomists, four cardiac vessels (namely, the vena cava, the artery-like vein, the vein-like artery, and the aorta or great artery) are united otherwise than they are in the adult.

The first contact and union is that of the vena cava with the vein-like artery. This takes place a little above the point where the cava emerges from the liver, and before it opens into the right ventricle, or gives off the coronary vein. The union results in a lateral anastomosis, that is, a large free opening, oval in shape, perforating from the cava into the artery in question. The opening is unimpeded, hence blood can pass very freely and abundantly through it (as through a single vessel) from the vena cava into the vein-like artery and the left auricle of the heart, and thence into the left ventricle. Further, there is in that oval opening, on the side facing the vein-like artery, a thin but strong membrane, like a lid, which is larger than the opening. Later on, in the adult, the membrane covers over the whole of this opening and, fusing with it at all points, renders it quite impervious and well-nigh effaces it. To revert, however, to the foetus – this membrane is so arranged that, in falling back loosely on itself, it moves easily in the direction of the lungs and the heart, and yields to the blood flowing against it from the cava but, on the other hand, prevents reflux of blood into that vessel. Hence, one may justifiably consider that in the embryo the blood must continuously be passing through this opening from the vena cava into the vein-like artery, and thence into the left auricle of the heart. On the other hand, once it has so entered, it can never flow back again.

The other union is of the artery-like vein (which occurs after that vein has left the right ventricle and is dividing into two branches). It is a sort of third trunk added to these two, an artery-like channel, so to speak, leading obliquely from this point to the great artery and perforating into it. Hence, in the dissection of embryos there appear, so to speak, to be two aortae, or two roots of the great artery arising from the heart. This channel, in the adult, narrows and dwindles in similar fashion to the foramen. Finally, it dries up internally like the umbilical vein, and ceases to exist.

The artery-like channel in question has no membrane inside it acting as an obstacle to the blood flow in either direction. For there are at the mouth of the artery-like vein (of which, as I have said, the channel in question is an offshoot) three sigmoid valves facing from within outwards. These yield easily to the blood flowing by this route from the right ventricle into the great artery, but completely prevent any reflux at all from the artery or from the lungs into the right ventricle, which they effectively shut off. Hence, in this instance also, it is proper to judge that in the embryo there is a continuous transference of blood by this route from the right ventricle into the great artery, during the contractions of the heart.

It is commonly said that these two unions, so large, free and open, have been made solely for the nutrition of the lungs: and that in the adult (though the lungs should now crave nutriment in greater amount because of their heat and movement) they cease to exist and are filled up. This is an objectionable and inconsistent fabrication. Equally false is the statement that in the embryo the heart is at rest, inactive and motionless, and that in consequence nature was forced to make these passages for the maintenance of the lungs. For one has only to look at an egg on which the hen has been sitting, and at embryos just removed from the uterus, to see quite clearly that the heart moves in them as in the adult, and that nature is under no such compulsion. I myself have often witnessed this movement, and the great Aristotle also testifies to it: 'The pulsation', he says, 'is evident from the very outset in the developing heart, as can be noticed in the dissection of living animals and in the growth of the chick from the egg.' Further, we see these routes (both in man and in other animals) open and free not only up to the time of birth (as anatomists have described) but even for many months after birth, nay in certain animals for a number of years, if not for the whole course of life, e.g. in the goose, snipe, and most birds, and in animals, particularly the smaller ones. It was this, perhaps, that misled Botallo into claiming that he had discovered a new passage for the blood from the vena cava into the left ventricle of the heart, and I confess that my own immediate reaction, on first finding this feature in a fairly large adult mouse, was somewhat similar.

These facts make it clear that there is absolute identity between what happens in the human embryo and what happens in others, in which the unions in question are not in the process of abolition. Hence the heart, by its movement, and through very patent pathways, transfers blood very obviously from the vena cava, through both ventricular conduits, into the great artery. The right ventricle receives blood from its auricle and then drives it forward through the artery-like vein and its offshoot (the so-called artery-like channel) into the great artery. The left ventricle, in like manner, simultaneously receives blood (that has been directed from the vena cava, by a different route, through the oval opening) by means of the auricular movement, and by its tension and constriction it drives this blood through the root of the aorta into the same great artery.

Thus in the embryo, while the lungs are idle and devoid of activity or movement, as though they did not exist, nature uses the two ventricles of the heart as one for the transmission of the blood. And the condition of the embryo that has lungs, but is not as yet making use of them, is similar to that of the animal that has no lungs at all.

The truth is thus as manifest in the foetus (as it is in the adult animal that has no lungs), namely, that the heart by its beat transfers blood from the vena cava and discharges it into the great artery. This it does by routes as free and open as would exist in man if the intervening septum were removed and the cavities of the two ventricles communicated with one another. Since, then, in the majority of animals at all times, and in all animals at some time, there exist such very wide ways for the passage of blood through the heart, it remains for us to make one or two inquiries. Either we should ask why in certain animals (as in man), and those warmer and full-grown, we believe no transfer takes place through the lung substance such as nature earlier effected in the embryo (at the time when the lungs were functionless) through ways which she appeared to have had to produce because of lack of a passage through the lungs. Alternatively, we should ask why it is advantageous that nature (who always does what is advantageous) has in adolescents completely closed to the passage of blood those widely open ways which she previously used in the embryo and foetus, and which she does [continuously] use in all other animals; why she has opened up no other ways for such passage of blood, but has in this manner produced a general hindrance to it.

The matter has thus got to the point that those who ask for the ways whereby in man the blood goes from the vena cava to the left ventricle and the vein-like artery would find it more rewarding and think it more satisfactory (supposing they wished to discover the truth from dissections of living animals) to inquire why in the larger and more perfect animals, and full-grown ones at that, nature should prefer the blood to be filtered through the lung parenchyma rather than, as in all other animal, through very wide ways (they would realize that these were the only alternative pathways). The answer may be as follows, or at least lie along some such lines. The larger and more perfect animals are naturally warmer and, when full-grown, can reasonably be described as over-heated and hard put to it to get rid of the excess. So the hot blood is carried to and through the lungs to be tempered by the inspired air and to be freed from bubbling to excess. But to settle these points and to give a full explanation is merely to explore the purpose of the lungs' fabrication. It is true that by very numerous observations I have discovered much about these organs and their function and movement, about ventilation as a whole, the need for and function of the air, the remaining kindred matters, and the various different organs produced in animals for this end. Nevertheless, lest I be thought to depart too greatly at this point from my main theme (the movement and function of the heart), and thereby to digress, leave my post, and confuse and evade the issue, I will leave these matters for more suitable exposition later in a special treatise. Those things which remain, to revert to my proposed object, I shall continue to establish.

I maintain that in the more perfect and warmer animals, and full-grown ones at that (as in man), the blood definitely permeates from the right ventricle of the heart through the artery-like vein into the lungs, thence through the vein-like artery into the left auricle, thence again into the left ventricle of the heart. I maintain, firstly, that this can happen; secondly, that it has so happened.

The blood permeates from the right ventricle of the heart through the parenchyma of the lungs into the vein-like artery and the left ventricle

We may agree that this can happen and that there is nothing to prevent it from happening when we think how water, permeating through the earth's substance, gives rise to streams and springs; or observe how sweats pass through the skin, or urine through the parenchyma of the kidneys. It is to be noted in those who use the waters of Spa, or the so-called waters of 'our Lady' in the Paduan countryside, or other waters of a mineral or sulphurous character, or in people who just measure their drink in gallons, that one to two hours suffice for them to pass it all out through the bladder as urine. The digestion of such a quantity must take a little while; and it must flow on through the liver (which all agree produces each day a double flow of juice from the food ingested), the veins, the parenchyma of the kidneys and the ureters into the bladder.

Whom then do I hear denying that blood, indeed, the whole mass of the blood, permeates through the substance of the lungs just as the juice of the food does through the liver, saying that such cannot happen, and must be regarded as altogether incredible? Such folk (in the words of the poet) allow readily that something can take place when they wish it so, but deny its possibility completely when they do not wish it so. They fear to assert it when it is necessary, and do not fear so when it is unnecessary.

The parenchyma of the liver is denser by far, and that of the kidneys likewise. That of the lungs is of much finer texture, and spongy by comparison with the kidneys and the liver. In the liver there is no inthrust, no driving force; in the lung, the blood is pushed in by the pulsation of the right ventricle of the heart, and by this inthrust the vessels and porosities of the lungs must be distended. Moreover, in breathing the lungs rise and fall, movement that necessitates the opening and closing respectively of the porosities and vessels; as happens in sponges, and in all parts having a spongy make-up, when they constrict and subsequently dilate. The liver, on the other hand, remains quiescent and has not been seen to dilate and constrict in this way.

Lastly, everyone agrees that the whole of the juice of the ingesta can pass through the liver into the vena cava in man as in the ox or in very large animals, and people have had to admit exactly this if nutriment is somehow to get through the liver to the veins for the purpose of nutrition and no other way is available. Why, in these circumstances, should they not have equal faith in the same proofs of the passage of blood through the lungs in these post-natal subjects, and assert and believe as did the very skilful and learned anatomist, Colombo, from the size and structure of the vessels of the lungs, and from the fact that the vein-like artery and likewise the ventricle are always full of blood which must have come to them through the veins and by no other path than an intrapulmonary one? He was, and we are, convinced of the truth of this by what has already been stated, by what has been seen in inspection of living animals, and by other proofs.

Since, however, there are some who defer only to duly adduced authorities, let these men know that this truth can be established from Galen's own words. Indeed, not only can blood pass from the artery-like vein into the vein-like artery and thence into the left ventricle of the heart and afterwards into the arteries, but this happens because of the continuous pulsations of the heart, and of the movement of the lungs in breathing.

[. . .] There is support for our claim that blood is continuously and unceasingly passing through the porosities of the lungs from the right to the left ventricle, from the vena cava into the aorta. For, as blood is continuously discharged from the right ventricle into the lungs through the artery-like vein, and is likewise continuously drawn from the lungs into the left ventricle (as is clear from what has been said, and from the position of the valves), it must continuously make the complete circuit.

In like manner, as blood is always continuously entering the right ventricle of the heart, and continuously emerging from the left one (as reason and sense alike show it to be), it cannot do other than pass right through from the vena cava into the aorta.

Thus that which dissection establishes as occurring through very wide passages in the majority of animals, and certainly in all animals before they are fully developed, is equally well established as occurring (according to Galen's statements and to what I have said above) in these fully developed animals through the invisible porosities of their lungs and the minute connections of the lung vessels. From which it is clear that one ventricle of the heart (namely, the left one) would suffice to distribute the blood through the body and to withdraw it from the vena cava (which indeed is the way it happens in all lungless creatures). When, however, nature wished the blood to be filtered through lungs, she was forced to make the extra provision of a right ventricle so that its pulsation would drive the blood through these very lungs from the vena cava to the region of the left ventricle. Thus one has to regard the right ventricle as having been made for the sake of the lungs and the transfer of blood, and not merely for nutrition. It is altogether incongruous to suppose that the lungs need for their nourishment so large a supply of food, so pulsatorily delivered, and also so much purer and more spirituous (as being supplied direct from the ventricles of the heart). For they cannot need such more than does the extremely pure substance of the brain, or the very fine and ineffable fabric of the eyes, or the flesh of the heart itself (which is more directly nourished through the coronary artery).

The amount of blood crossing through the heart from the veins into the arteries; the circular movement of the blood

Thus far I have written about the transfer of blood from the veins into the arteries, the paths through which such crossing is effected, and the manner in which the blood is transmitted and distributed as a result of the heart's pulsation. In respect of which matters there are perhaps some who, after my recalling of Galen's authoritative statements or the reasonings of Colombo or of others, may say that they are in agreement with me. The remaining matters, however (namely, the amount and source of the blood which so crosses through from the veins into the arteries), though well worthy of consideration, are so novel and hitherto unmentioned that, in speaking of them, I not only fear that I may suffer from the ill-will of a few, but dread lest all men turn against me. To such an extent is it virtually second nature for all to follow accepted usage and teaching which, since its first implanting, has become deep-rooted; to such extent are men swayed by a pardonable respect for the ancient authors. However, the die has now been cast, and my hope lies in the love of truth and the clear-sightedness of the trained mind. In attempting to discover how much blood passes from the veins into the arteries I made dissections of living animals, opened up arteries in them, and carried out various other investigations. I also considered the symmetry and size of the ventricles of the heart and of the vessels which enter and leave them (since nature, who does nothing purposelessly, would not purposelessly have given these vessels such relatively large size). I also recalled the elegant and carefully contrived valves and fibres and other structural artistry of the heart; and many other points. I considered rather often and with care all this evidence, and took correspondingly long trying to assess how much blood was transmitted and in how short a time. I also noted that the juice of the ingested food could not supply this amount without our having the veins, on the one hand, completely emptied and the arteries, on the other hand, brought to bursting through excessive inthrust of blood, unless the blood somehow flowed back again from the arteries into the veins and returned to the right ventricle of the heart. In consequence, I began privately to consider if it had a movement, as it were, in a circle. This hypothesis I subsequently verified, finding that the pulsation of the left ventricle of the heart forces the blood out of it and propels it through the arteries into all parts of the body's system in exactly the same way as the pulsation of the right ventricle forces the blood out of that chamber and propels it through the artery-like vein into the lungs; finding, further, that the blood flows back again through the veins and the vena cava and right up to the right auricle in exactly the same way as it flows back from the lungs through the so-called vein-like artery to the left ventricle (as already described).

We have as much right to call this movement of the blood circular as Aristotle had to say that the air and rain emulate the circular movement of the heavenly bodies. The moist earth, he wrote, is warmed by the sun and gives off vapours which condense as they are carried up aloft and in their condensed form fall again as rain and remoisten the earth, so producing successions of fresh life from it. In similar fashion the circular movement of the sun, that is to say, its approach and recession, give rise to storms and atmospheric phenomena.

It may very well happen thus in the body with the movement of the blood. All parts may be nourished, warmed, and activated by the hotter, perfect, vaporous, spirituous and, so to speak, nutritious blood. On the other hand, in parts the blood may be cooled, coagulated and be figuratively worn out. From such parts it returns to its starting-point, namely, the heart, as if to its source or to the centre of the body's economy, to be restored to its erstwhile state of perfection. Therein, by the natural, powerful, fiery heat, a sort of store of life, it is re-liquefied and becomes impregnated with spirits and (if I may so style it) sweetness. From the heart it is redistributed. And all these happenings are dependent upon the pulsatile movement of the heart.

This organ deserves to be styled the starting point of life and the sun of our microcosm just as much as the sun deserves to be styled the heart of the world. For it is by the heart's vigorous beat that the blood is moved, perfected, activated, and protected from injury and coagulation. The heart is the tutelary deity of the body, the basis of life, the source of all things, carrying out its function of nourishing, warming, and activating the body as a whole. But we shall more fittingly speak of these matters when we consider the final cause of this kind of movement.

To conclude, though veins are precise channels and vessels for the carriage of blood, they are two kinds, the cava and the aorta, not because these lie on opposite sides of the body (Aristotle's view) but by virtue of difference in function, and not (as commonly held) because they are structurally dissimilar (since in many animals, as I have stated above, a vein does not differ from an artery in the thickness of its coat) but because they are distinct from each other in office and usage. Though vein and artery were not unreasonably both styled veins (as Galen noted) by the ancients, one of them, namely the artery, is a vessel which carries blood from the heart to the component parts of the body, while the other is a vessel which carries blood from those component parts back to the heart. The one is a channel from, the other a channel to, the heart. The latter channel contains cruder, worn-out blood that has been returned unfit for nutrition; the former contains mature, perfected, nutritive blood.

The existence of a circuit of the blood proved by confirmation of the first supposition

But lest anyone say that we cheat and merely make plausible assertions without a basis and advance new views without just cause, there are three suppositions which come up for confirmation. If these are stated, then I think the truth which I advocate automatically follows and the fact is plain to all.

The first supposition is that the blood is continuously and uninterruptedly transmitted by the beat of the heart from the vena cava into the arteries in such amount that it cannot be supplied from the ingesta, and thus in such wise that the whole mass of the blood passes across from the vena cava into the arteries within a short space of time.

The second supposition is that the blood is continuously, evenly, and uninterruptedly driven by the beat of the arteries into every member and part, entering each in far greater amount than is sufficient for its nutrition or can be supplied to it [without such rapid circular movement] by the whole mass of the blood.

The third supposition, similarly, is that the veins themselves are constantly returning this blood from each and every member to the region of the heart.

With these suppositions thus stated, I think it will be manifest that the blood goes round and is returned, is driven forward and flows back, from the heart to the extremities, and thence back again to the heart, and so executes a sort of circular movement.
[. . .]

Conclusion of my description of the circuit of the blood

May I now be permitted to summarize my view about the circuit of the blood, and to make it generally known!

Since calculations and visual demonstrations have confirmed all my suppositions, to wit, that the blood is passed through the lungs and the heart by the pulsation of the ventricles, is forcibly ejected to all parts of the body, therein steals into the veins and the porosities of the flesh, flows back everywhere through those very veins from the circumference to the centre, from small veins into larger ones, and thence comes at last into the vena cava and to the auricle of the heart; all this, too, in such amount and with so large a flux and reflux – from the heart out to the periphery, and back from the periphery to the heart – that it cannot be supplied from the ingesta, and is also in much greater bulk than would suffice for nutrition.

I am obliged to conclude that in animals the blood is driven round a circuit with an unceasing, circular sort of movement, that this is an activity or function of the heart which it carries out by virtue of its pulsation, and that in sum it constitutes the sole reason for that heart's pulsatile movement.

Part Three **Development**

Thomas Sydenham

Those who called Thomas Sydenham 'the English Hippocrates' paid him a great compliment: they were declaring that Sydenham manifested the great virtues of the Father of Medicine. Hippocrates had relied on careful observation and cautious inference which did not outrun the observable facts. At the opposite extreme was the theorist who indulged in theoretical elaborations and gave logical priority to the ultimate constituents of the universe, the primary metaphysical 'building blocks'. Such a theorist could then fit the data of medicine into a system of which these abstractions formed the base. Sydenham, like Hippocrates, placed observation above theory.

In the seventeenth century the Galenic tradition had become bogged down in logical subtleties and fine-spun distinctions that were so brilliantly satirized by Molière. At the same time new theory, derived from the mechanical philosophy on the one hand, from the chemical philosophers on the other, was attracting attention and exerting great influence. But much of the influence was on the theoretical level, involving the formation of hypotheses. Sydenham wanted to return to the old tradition of medical practice founded on direct observation of the patient. He had little sympathy with the newer 'natural philosophy' which had not really advanced the concrete care of the patient.

Sydenham was born in 1624. His university education was interrupted by the Civil War, in which he supported the parliamentary faction. He did receive his bachelor of medicine degree at Oxford, but his training was markedly curtailed and severely inadequate, even by the standards of the day. He did not have the traditional classical background that characterized seventeenth-century university education in England at that time, but relied more on his own powers of observation and strong native intelligence.

His first medical publication, and one of his most important writings, was the *Medical Observations Concerning the History and Cure of Acute Diseases* (1666). In the preface to the enlarged third edition (1676), Sydenham indicated the main principles of his methodology. Our quotations are taken from this preface.

Sydenham stressed the importance of natural history – the accurate and impartial description of the phenomena of nature, in as great detail as possible, without theoretical elaboration or interpretation. Diseases, as phenomena of nature, had for him a reality comparable to the reality of plants; and like plants, diseases should be classified according to their essential features.

The phenomena of disease included not only the manifestations or symptoms but also the reactions of the patients to various medications. However, it was not enough merely to record the disease and the means of combating these diseases successfully through medicine. Such a procedure was the province of the 'empiric', the untutored person who did not understand the workings of nature but practised without any knowledge of reasons and causes. Sydenham emphasized the necessity for understanding the causes of phenomena, for without such knowledge of causes any medical practice is blind. But he strongly insisted that the search for causes should be limited to observable phenomena, and he condemned the flights to abstractions that lay beyond direct experience.

Subsequent developments in methodology and philosophy of science have shown that Sydenham was quite naïve in his approach to medical science, but he did exert great and much-needed influence as a counterweight to the speculative tendencies prevalent at this time. And his insistence on observation and cautious inference helped to lay the foundations for the great subsequent development of medicine.

7 Medical Observations (1676)

Excerpts from Thomas Sydenham, 'Medical Observations concerning the History and Cure of Acute Diseases [3rd edn, 1676]', in *The Works of Thomas Sydenham*, translated by R. G. Latham, vol. 1, The Sydenham Society, 1848, pp. 11–21.

[. . .]

5. I conceive that the advancement of medicine lies in the following conditions:

There must be, in the first place, a history of the disease; in other words, a description that shall be at once graphic and natural.

There must be, in the second place, a *Praxis*, or *Methodus*, respecting the same, and this must be regular and exact.

To draw a disease in gross is an easy matter. To describe it in its history, so as to escape the censure of the great Bacon, is far more difficult. Against some pretenders in this way, he launches the following censure:

We are well aware that there existeth such a thing as a Natural History; full in bulk, pleasant from its variety, often curious from its diligence. Notwithstanding, whoever would take away from the same the citations of authors, the empty discussions, and, finally, the book-learning and ornaments, which are fitter for the convivial meetings of learned men than for the establishment of a Philosophy, would find that it dwindled into nothing. Such a natural history is far distant from the one we contemplate.

In like manner it is exceedingly easy to propound some commonplace cure for a complaint. It is far harder, however, to translate your words into actions, and to square your results with your promises. This is well known to those who have learned that there occur in practical writers numerous diseases, which neither the authors themselves, nor any persons else besides, have been able to cure.

6. In respect to the histories of a disease, any one who looks at the case carefully, will see at once that an author must direct his attention to many more points than are usually thought of. A few of these are all that need be noticed at present.

7. In the first place, it is necessary that all diseases be reduced

to definite and certain *species*, and that, with the same care which we see exhibited by botanists in their phytologies; since it happens, at present, that many diseases, although included in the same genus, mentioned with a common nomenclature, and resembling one another in several symptoms, are, notwithstanding, different in their natures, and require a different medical treatment.

We all know that the term *thistle* is applied to a variety of plants; nevertheless, he would be a careless botanist, indeed, who contented himself with the general description of a *thistle*; who only exhibited the marks by which the class was identified; who neglected the proper and peculiar signs of the species, and who overlooked the characters by which they were distinguished from each other. On the same principle, it is not enough for a writer to merely note down the common phenomena of some multiform disease; for, although it may be true that all complaints are not liable to the same amount of variety, there are still many which authors treat alike, under the same heads, and without the shadows of a distinction, whilst they are in their nature as dissimilar as possible. This I hope to prove in the forthcoming pages.

8. More than this – it generally happens that even where we find a *specific* distribution, it has been done in subservience to some favourite hypothesis which lies at the bottom of the true phenomena; so that the distinction has been adapted not to the nature of the complaint, but to the views of the author and the character of his philosophy. Many instances prove the extent to which medicine has been injured by a want of accuracy upon this point. We should have known the cures of many diseases before this time if physicians, whilst with all due goodwill they communicated their experiments and observations, had not been deceived in their disease, and had not mistaken one species for another. And this, I think, is one reason why the *Materia Medica* has grown so much and produced so little.

9. In writing the history of a disease, every philosophical hypothesis whatsoever, that has previously occupied the mind of the author, should lie in abeyance. This being done, the clear and natural phenomena of the disease should be noted – these, and these only. They should be noted accurately, and in all their

minuteness; in imitation of the exquisite industry of those painters who represent in their portraits the smallest moles and the faintest spots. No man can state the errors that have been occasioned by these physiological hypotheses. Writers, whose minds have taken a false colour under their influence, have saddled diseases with phenomena which existed in their own brains only; but which would have been clear and visible to the whole world had the assumed hypothesis been true. Add to this, that if by chance some symptom really coincide accurately with their hypothesis, and occur in the disease whereof they would describe the character, they magnify it beyond all measure and moderation; they make it all and in all; the molehill becomes a mountain; whilst, if it fail to tally with the said hypothesis, they pass it over either in perfect silence or with only an incidental mention, unless, by means of some philosophical subtlety, they can enlist it in their service, or else, by fair means or foul, accommodate it in some way or other to their doctrines.

10. Thirdly; it is necessary, in describing any disease, to enumerate the peculiar and constant phenomena apart from the accidental and adventitious ones: these last-named being those that arise from the age or temperament of the patient, and from the different forms of medical treatment. It often happens that the character of the complaint varies with the nature of the remedies, and that symptoms may be referred less to the disease than to the doctor. Hence two patients with the same ailment, but under different treatment, may suffer from different symptoms. Without caution, therefore, our judgment concerning the symptoms of disease is, of necessity, vague and uncertain. Outlying forms of disease, and cases of exceeding rarity, I take no notice of. They do not properly belong to the histories of disease. No botanist takes the bites of a caterpillar as a characteristic of a leaf of sage.

11. Finally, the particular seasons of the year which favour particular complaints are carefully to be observed. I am ready to grant that many diseases are good for all seasons. On the other hand, there is an equal number that, through some mysterious instinct of nature, follow the seasons as truly as plants and birds of passage. I have often wondered that this disposition on the part of several diseases, obvious as it is, has been so little observed;

the more so, as there is no lack of curious observations upon the planets under which plants grow and beasts propagate. But whatever may be the cause of this supineness, I lay it down as a confirmed rule, that the knowledge of the seasons wherein diseases occur is of equal value to the physician in determining their species and in effecting their extirpation; and that both these results are less satisfactory when this observation is neglected.

12. These, although not the only, are the main points to be attended to in drawing up the history of a disease. The practical value of such a history is above all calculation. By the side thereof, the subtle discussions, and the minute refinements wherewith the books of our new school are stuffed full, even *ad nauseam*, are of no account. What short way – what way at all – is there towards either the detection of the morbific cause that we must fight against, or towards the indications of treatment which we must discover, except the sure and distinct perception of peculiar symptoms? Upon each of these points the slightest and most unimportant circumstances have their proper bearings. Something in the way of variety we may refer to the particular temperament of individuals; something also to the difference of treatment. Notwithstanding this, nature, in the production of disease, is uniform and consistent; so much so, that for the same disease in different persons the symptoms are for the most part the same; and the selfsame phenomena that you would observe in the sickness of a Socrates you would observe in the sickness of a simpleton. Just so the universal characters of a plant are extended to every individual of the species; and whoever (I speak in the way of illustration) should accurately describe the colour, the taste, the smell, the figure, etc., of one single violet, would find that his description held good, there or thereabouts, for all the violets of that particular species upon the face of the earth.

13. For my own part, I think that we have lived thus long without an accurate history of diseases, for this especial reason viz. that the generality have considered that disease is but a confused and disordered effort of nature thrown down from her proper state, and defending herself in vain; so that they have classed the attempts at a just description with the attempts to wash blackamoors white.

14. To return, however, to our business. As truly as the

physician may collect points of diagnosis from the minutest circumstances of the disease, so truly may he also elicit indications in the way of therapeutics. So much does this statement hold good, that I have often thought, that provided with a thorough insight into the history of any disease whatsoever, I could invariably apply an equivalent remedy; a clear path being thus marked out for me by the different phenomena of the complaint. These phenomena, if carefully collated with each other, lead us, as it were, by the hand to those palpable indications of treatment which are drawn, not from the hallucinations of our fancy, but from the innermost penetralia of nature.

15. By this ladder, and by this scaffold, did Hippocrates ascend his lofty sphere – the Romulus of medicine, whose heaven was the empyrean of his art. He it is whom we can never duly praise. He it was who then laid the solid and immoveable foundation for the whole superstructure of medicine, when he taught that *our natures are the physicians of our diseases*. By this he ensured a clear record of the phenomena of each disease, pressing into his service no hypothesis, and doing no violence to his description; [. . .].

Now, as the said theory was neither more nor less than an exquisite picture of nature, it was natural that the practice should coincide with it. This aimed at one point only – it strove to help nature in her struggles as it best could. With this view, it limited the province of medical art to the support of nature when she was enfeebled, and to the coercion of her when she was outrageous; the attempt on either side being determined by the rate and method whereby she herself attempted the removal and the expulsion of disease. The great sagacity of this man had discovered that nature by herself *determines diseases, and is of herself sufficient in all things against all of them*. This she is, being aided by the fewest and the simplest forms of medicine. At times she is independent of even these.

16. The other method whereby, in my opinion, the art of medicine may be advanced, turns chiefly upon what follows, viz. that there must be some fixed, definite, and consummate *methodus medendi*, of which the commonweal may have the advantage. By *fixed*, *definite*, and *consummate*, I mean a line of practice which has been based and built upon a sufficient number

of experiments, and has in that manner been proved competent to the cure of this or that disease. I by no means am satisfied with the record of a few successful operations, either of the doctor or the drug. I require that they be shown to succeed universally, or at least under such and such circumstances. [. . .]

I am far from denying that a physician ought to attend diligently to particular cases in respect to the results both of the method and of the remedies which he employs in the cure of disease. I grant, too, that he may lay up his experiences for use, both in the way of easing his memory and of seizing suggestions. By so doing he may gradually increase in medical skill, so that eventually, by a long continuance and a frequent repetition of his experiments, he may lay down and prescribe for himself a *methodus medendi*, from which, in the cure of this or that disease, he need not deviate a single straw's breadth.

17. Nevertheless, the publication of particular observations is, in my mind, of no great advantage. Where is the particular importance in just telling us that once, twice or even oftener, this disease has yielded to that remedy? We are overwhelmed as it is, with an infinite abundance of vaunted medicaments, and here they add a new one. Now, if I repudiate the rest of my formulae, and restrict myself to this medicine only, I must try its efficacy by innumerable experiments, and I must weigh, in respect to both the patient and the practice, innumerable circumstances, before I can derive any benefit from such a solitary observation.

But if the medicine never fails in the hands of the observer, why does he confine himself to particular cases? He must either distrust himself, or he must desire to impose upon the world in detail, rather than in gross. How easy a matter it is to write thick volumes upon these points is known even to beginners. It is also known that the foundation and erection of a perfect and definite *methodus medendi* is a work of exceeding difficulty. If, in each age of the world, a single person only had properly treated upon one single disease, the province of the physician, or the art of healing, would long ago have reached its height; and would have been as complete and perfect as the lot of humanity admits. It is ruin of our prospects to have departed from our oldest and best guide, Hippocrates, and to have forsaken the original *methodus medendi*. This was built upon the knowledge of immediate and conjunct causes, things of which the evidence is certain. Our modern doctrine is a contrivance of the word-catchers; the art of talking rather than the art of healing.

That I may not seem to speak these things rashly, I must be allowed to make a brief digression; and to prove that those remote and ultimate causes in the determination and exhibition of which the vain speculations of curious and busy men are solely engaged, are altogether incomprehensible and inscrutable; and that the only causes that can be known to us, and the only ones from which we may draw our indications of treatment, are those which are proximate, immediate, and conjunct.

[. . .]

19. Let a person seriously and accurately consider the phenomena which accompany such a fever as a quartan ague. It begins almost always in autumn; it keeps to a regular course of succession; it preserves a definite type; its periodical revolutions, occurring on the fourth day, if undisturbed by external influences, are as regular as those of a watch or any other piece of machinery; it sets in with shivers and a notable feeling of cold, which are succeeded by an equally decided sensation of heat, and it is terminated by a most profuse perspiration. Whoever is attacked must bear with his complaint till the vernal equinox, there or therabouts.

Now putting all this carefully together, we find reasons for believing that this disease is a species equally cogent with those that we have for believing a plant to be a species. The plant springs from the earth; the plant blooms; the plant dies: the plant does all this with equal regularity. [. . .]

20. Now, although it appears, from what has been said, that we have shown reason for considering the causes of the majority of diseases as inscrutable and inexplicable, the question as to how they may be cured is, nevertheless, capable of solution.

All that we have just dealt with has been the case of the remote causes. Here it is evident to every one, that curious speculators lose their labour; since the investigation and illustration of primary and ultimate causes is a neglect of our capabilities, and a violation of nature. Hand in hand with this is the contempt for those causes that ought to be, and which can be understood; which lie before our feet; which require no rotten supports; which appeal to the understanding at once; which are revealed by either the testimony of our senses, or by anatomical observations of long standing. Such are the causes which we call conjunct and immediate. As it is clearly impossible that a physician should discover those causes of disease that are not cognizable by the senses, so also it is unnecessary that he should attempt it. It is quite sufficient for him to know whence the mischief *immediately* arises, and for him to be able to distinguish with accuracy between the effects and symptoms of the complaint which he has in hand, and those of some similar one. In a pleurisy, for instance, a man may work much, and work in vain, before he will understand the vicious crasis, and the incoherent texture of blood which is the primary cause of the disease; yet, if he know rightly the cause by which it is *immediately* produced, and if he can rightly discriminate between it and other diseases, he will be as certain to succeed in his attempts at a cure, as if he had attended to idle and unprofitable searches into remote causes.

Friederich Hoffmann

Friederich Hoffmann (1660–1742), one of the great systematists of the eighteenth century, was a prolific writer who exerted a considerable influence on the medicine of his era, primarily on the continent and to a lesser degree in England. For our purposes one of his early writings, never previously translated into English, has particular significance. This book, whose Anglicized title would be *The Foundations of Medicine*, he published in 1695, shortly after he was appointed professor of medicine at the newly founded University of Halle. He gave an epitome of medical doctrine, in short aphoristic paragraphs which, in the aggregate, supply a compendium of medicine. The book, in five sections, covers physiology, pathology, semeiology (diagnosis), hygiene and therapeutics. The presentation is dogmatic, offering assertions and conclusions without supporting evidence. The quotations here given (my own translation from the original Latin) illustrate the systematic presentation of medical theory and the 'rationalistic' approach that contrasts with the empirical attitudes of Sydenham.

Writing in the rationalistic tradition, he began with basic constituents and principles, discussing matter and motion, body and mind and, by implication if not by direct statement, the metaphysical foundations of medical science. A rapid transition to the principles of physics and chemistry then provided the basis of physiology and pathology, and following this he discussed the states of health and disease.

Serving as the basis for lectures, a book such as this illustrates rationalistic medicine at the end of the seventeenth century. There was no attempt to provide valid evidence to prove a point. Indeed, the whole notion of proof as we understand it had no place in the presentation. Instead, the logical interrelation between a given assertion and the basic premises was considered an adequate demonstration. As we read these selections we see the complete dogmatism, the reliance on definitions and on inferences from the definitions, and the assertion of hypotheses as if they were actual facts. To be sure, all the statements ultimately rested on some sort of observation or experiment, but the question whether the observational evidence was reliable or whether it could support the inferences drawn, did not arise.

The few excerpts indicate the rationalist methodology, and in addition give some indication of the various doctrinal components. Galenic teachings persisted along with the newer concepts of the circulation and other physiological discoveries. To this mixture the mechanical philosophy and iatrochemistry both made contributions, and a suggestion of Cartesian metaphysics permeates the whole.

The short excerpts do not give a systematic exposition of Hoffmann's teachings, but they suffice to indicate the mechanistic viewpoint. The body was considered to be a machine composed of fluid parts and solid parts, and its workings in both health and disease could be understood by understanding the motion of particulate matter. Mechanics and hydrodynamics were the important subjects. There were many kinds of material particles and they had different chemical properties. Such properties, however, were conceived in mechanical terms, and chemical attraction was considered, in essence, a mechanical process.

8 Foundations of Medicine (1695)

Excerpts from Friederich Hoffmann, *Fundamenta medicinae*, translated by Lester S. King, MacDonald and Elsevier, 1971, pp. 5–60.

Book I Physiology

Chapter 1: Of the nature of medicine

1. Medicine is the art of properly utilizing physico-mechanical principles, in order to conserve the health of man or to restore it if lost.

[. . .]

6. The physician is the servant of nature, not her master; the principles of nature and of art are the same and hence the physician must work and act with nature.

7. In medicine there are two supports – experience, which is the first parent of truth; and reason, which is the key to medical science. Experience comes first in order, and reason follows. Hence in medical affairs reasons which are not founded on experience have no value.

8. In physics, experience can best be sought from mathematics and mechanics, chemistry and anatomy; in medical practice, experience derives most abundantly from the observations of diseases, and from more accurate histories and cures.

9. As far as medicine uses the principles of physics it can be properly called a science; as far as it relies on practice, it can be called an art.

10. The perfect physician must have not only the knowledge of medical art, but also prudence and wisdom.

[. . .]

Chapter 2: Of the mechanico-physical principles of things

1. Like all of nature, medicine must be mechanical.

2. The first principles of mechanics are matter and motion; therefore, the elements thought up by the peripatetics and the chemists are mere imaginings.

3. The essence of matter is seen to consist in extension. From this derives finitude, shape, divisibility, and impenetrability.

4. Motion is the first and most universal principle of things and

the efficient cause of all forms. As matter gives the essence common to all things, so motion provides them with specificity.

5. Matter differs in regard to shape as well as size. It can best be divided in a threefold fashion: an extremely subtle matter, a subtle or ethereal matter, and a more dense or earthy and aqueous form.

6. All bodies are observed as either solid or fluid. The cause of fluidity are the two first elements, and of solidity, the last.

7. All natural bodies are put together out of this threefold matter; and the forms and qualities of bodies vary, as particles differ in shape and extension and are skillfully combined with each other in a certain order.

8. There are no substantial forms, but all of these represent accidents in respect to matter, although they can be called essential, in regard to structure. [. . .]

9. Size, shape, motion and rest are entire basic states of simple bodies. From these, therefore, the reasons for all natural phenomena and effects are to be sought.

10. God is the first cause of all motion, and also of all forms. Matter, which is purely passive, necessarily requires a certain agent which differentiated it into the very many different forms that constitute the world; or which divided that extension into various parts, moulded, moved and transposed it. This principle is God alone.

[. . .]

Chapter 3: Of health, life, proportion and nature

1. Our body is like a machine or automaton whose organs, varying in shape and size, are disposed and constructed in a particular order and position. These organs must be moved and animated by the fluid parts of our body.

2. The parts of our body are either solid or fluid. If the fluids are constituted in a suitable proportion and have an equable motion, and the solids exist in a suitable configuration, position and order, the body is then suited to exert its functions according to nature, and is healthy.

[. . .]

4. The life of the body consists in the continuous and appropriate movement of the fluid parts through the solids. The fluid

parts, moreover, are the primary cause of motion, and they excite the solids into motion.

[. . .]

7. Life is achieved by causes which are wholly mechanical. The mind does not bring life to the body, nor is life oriented to the mind, but rather to the body.

8. When a human body dies it is not the mind that recedes from the body; rather the body recedes from the mind, since the organs of the body have become corrupt, so that the mind can no longer preside over them.

9. Just as life consists in motion of the fluid parts and health in well-ordered and even motion, so death is only a destruction of motion, or motion disproportionate and uneven.

10. It is not the solid parts, considered in themselves, that can be said to be well ordered or disordered, but their due proportion depends on the proportion and motion of the fluid parts.

11. When the different small particles constituting the blood – earthy, branching, watery, saline, volatile, fixed, acid or sulphurous – are intermixed in a proportionate fashion, so that they bring about an even motion among themselves, then the blood is considered properly mixed [*temperatus*] and a smooth proportion [*blanda temperies*] is introduced into the solid parts.

12. The more unevenly these small bodies are mixed the more there results an uneven motion and varied disproportion.

13. When sulphurous, oily, volatile or saline particles predominate over the fixed, or watery, or earthy ones, the disproportion is *warm*, and then the resulting temperament is called warm or sanguine; and if the excess is too great, then a choleric temperament results.

14. We say that a person has a warm temperament who is composed of such a fibrous plexus, in which many warm ethereal, fiery particles are present, or in which many such particles can easily aggregate together.

15. But if the watery mucilaginous acid fixed particles predominate over the sulphurous, spirituous or saline ones of the blood, there arises a phlegmatic, cold-moist temperament. And when those particles are accompanied by acid salts, it is called melancholy, which differs merely in grade from phlegmatic.

16. We call phlegmatic those who abound in serous humours,

and are composed of a plexus of fibres so dense that the warm parts can be concentrated only with difficulty.

17. In the sanguine and choleric temperament the motion of the fluid parts is more vigorous, rapid, and swift; in the phlegmatic, however, and the melancholic, it is more slow and diminished.

18. The motion of the animal spirits is dependent on the proper mixture and motion of the blood and the humours; and the motions of the mind, its inclinations and thoughts arise in proportion to the motion and proper mixture of the animal spirits. Hence, as Galen said, the habits of the mind follow the temperament of the body.

[. . .]

Chapter 4: Of the solid and fluid parts of the human machine, especially of the blood

24. The solid components of the living body are entirely tubular. That the most minute parts are hollow is proved by the circulation of blood in the louse, and through the tail fibrils in the eel. This can best be demonstrated by the microscope.

25. The solid parts, since they are woven together out of innumerable extremely minute threads and fibrils, must have many thousands of intermediate spaces, or intervals between the small bodies out of which they are aggregated.

26. Most important of the fluid parts is the blood mass, composed of innumerable particles and small bodies, differing in size, shape and weight.

27. In the blood there lie hidden many kinds of particles – serous, slippery, flexible and rigid, saline, both volatile and acid, branching, sulphurous, oily, dense, mucilaginous, and earthy.

[. . .]

37. The blood enjoys a twofold motion. One, internal, is of the smallest particles reciprocally with each other; and the other is circulatory or progressive, by means of which blood is carried through the vessels. Neither can exist without the other.

38. Each of these motions is due to the elastic power of the air and ether, communicated through respiration, and to the vigour and motion of the heart.

39. The motion of the heart takes place by contraction or sys-

tole, and dilatation or diastole. The heart is not so much the workshop as the bellows of the blood, serving to receive it and expel it.

40. The heart is nothing but a muscle, constructed in geometric fashion of fibres and moving fibrous threads and suitable for vigorous contraction and dilatation.

41. The heart is the first principle of all motion in our body and of the circulation of the blood (without which man cannot live); it is the instrument and the prime force impelling the blood.

42. The motion of the heart is not due to any innate motor power, but to the expansive effort of the spirituous seminal fluid in the embryo itself. In adults it seems due to the expansive force of the ether and of animal spirits and blood.

[. . .]

Chapter 6: Of the vital motion of our machine, and sensation

1. Nothing in the microcosmic machine is performed without motion; no change, secretion, nutrition, or sensation can occur without motion.

2. The fluid parts move. Among these the nerve fluid demands first place, for it is the finest of all and most suited for producing very rapid movement. On it depend the motion of all the parts of the machine, both solid and fluid.

3. The animal spirits, provided with the utmost fineness and elasticity, have a power impressed by God, not only of moving themselves mechanically, but doing so by choice, purposefully [*determinate*] and towards a definite goal. This power is called the sensitive soul, and it exists entirely in the most subtle fluid of the brain.

4. The motor fibres, and their various intertwinings and interweavings, are the organic instrument of movement of the animal fluids.

5. When the motor fibres are so interwoven among themselves that the two extremities become tendons while the middle part is more loose, we then have a muscle, which is the instrument of voluntary motion.

6. When motor fibres are layered upon themselves in a certain definite order, some of them transversely, we have a muscular or fleshy membrane which is the organ of involuntary and natural motion.

7. We can see for ourselves that there exists a muscular tunic of the stomach, intestines, urinary bladder, biliary passages, ureters, arteries and veins, which has fleshy and motor fibres intertwined with each other.

8. The animal spirits, by their mobile and expansive nature, flow into the fibres, and thus shorten and distend them, so that what they give up in length, they acquire in thickness. Of course, the configuration but not the mass is changed as the muscle swells.

[. . .]

Chapter 7: Of the function of the viscera, animal secretion and nutrition

20. The blood has not only a progressive and circulatory motion but an internal one. The internal motion is prior to the circulatory and on this internal motion depends the formation of spirits, strength and energy itself.

21. The motion of the blood is maintained by subtle particles of elastic air, which, by virtue of shape and size, bring about a certain vital swelling in various particles of the blood. On this swelling depend the energy of the body and at the same time the motion of the heart itself.

22. The ethereal elastic particles drawn in by respiration cannot bring about the vital swellings, if the blood is too thick and abounds in fixed particles or if it is too fluid, expanded and fine. Hence, strength requires well ordered blood.

23. Not only the heart but the arteries themselves, the veins, even all the vessels, viscera and muscles contribute to the progressive and the local motion of the blood, and can increase or diminish this, render it even or uneven.

[. . .]

31. The vesicles of the lungs serve for the finer segregation of the aereal particles which get intermixed with the blood. Furthermore, the coarser aqueous particles are again thrown out through expiration.

32. The more subtle portion of the air, endowed with elastic force, divides the globules of the blood and drives them apart, produces motion or internal fermentation, fluidity, vital heat and a purplish colour.

33. The air does not cool, but makes warm. Hence the more rapid is inspiration, as in motion and in exercise, the greater is the heat that is present.

[. . .]

35. The animal spirits and the nutrient juice have their origin from blood mixed with serum. Nature especially intends the production of these fluids from the blood, and to this end harmoniously blends the functions of all viscera.

36. Our nutrient juice, whose very fine volatile parts furnish the material for these animal spirits, should consist of globular fluid particles, sweet, gelatinous and properly mixed.

37. The particles that are more viscid and fixed, acid, saline, sulphurous, sharp, cannot enter into the production of the nutrient juice and the material of the animal spirits.

38. The functions of almost all the viscera combine to the end that the saline, more rigid, earthy and viscid particles should be separated from the blood and serum, and the coarser ones be made finer.

39. The viscera do not separate out the excremental humours through any ferment that precipitates the humours to be secreted, but all secretion of the bile, urine, sweat, phlegm, saliva, is accomplished by mechanical means and a particular manner of filtration.

40. The glandular pores and vessels of the liver separate from the blood the bitter sulphurous particles which, collected in the gall bladder, constitute the bile.

41. The kidneys, which consist of extremely fine canaliculi, filter from the blood the salt serum which is called urine.

42. The very minute vessels, glands, and pores of the skin separate off that vaporous salt serum which goes by the name of sweat.

[. . .]

Book II Medical pathology

Chapter 1: Of diseases in general and their causes

1. Life and health consist in the proper functioning of the vital actions: disease, in the distorted or diminished functioning; and death, in its total destruction.

2. When the vital actions, involved in the movement, sensation

and nutrition of the machine, are injured, then disease, or an abnormal disposition of our machine is said to be present.

3. As the vital actions depend directly on the proper laudable, and even motion of the fluid parts, especially the animal spirits, and the proper conformation of the solids, diminished and distorted vital actions arise from the impaired motions of the humours and the distorted conformation of the solids.

4. Death takes place when the proportion and movement of the fluids constituting our machine are totally destroyed. The greater the degree of destruction affecting the proportion or motion of the humours, the more severe and dangerous is the disease.

5. Whatever injures or destroys the proportion and the laudable motion of the blood and nerve fluid, or the configuration of the solid parts (which consists in proper situation, number and shape) deserves the title of morbific cause.

6. Disproportion does not affect the solid parts except as it is derived from the fluid parts. [. . .]

7. Abnormal disposition and weakness of the viscera consists in the changing state of pores and tubules and in obstruction.

8. A disproportion of the fluid parts results from the impaired mixture of their constituent particles.

9. The fluid parts consist of particles varying in respect to mass, shape and position; if the volatile, fluid and spirituous particles, and those that are fixed, earthy, and mucilaginous, are correctly mixed with each other and reach an equilibrium, then a due proportion is present; and on the contrary, if this mixture is uneven, then a disproportion results.

10. Disproportions can best be referred to two categories. Either the mobile, volatile, saline, and sulphurous particles predominate in the blood and humours, and then a disproportion arises that is warm, saline and sharp; or else the mucilaginous, acid and fixed particles predominate, and then a disproportion results that is cold, acid, and melancholic.

[. . .]

Chapter 2: Of the remote causes of diseases

1. The parentage, nativity, and the land, the age, sex and mode of life are relevant [*faciunt*] to the proportion and natural constitution of the blood and nerve fluid, and to health itself. These also

can take part in the disproportion of the blood and the production of diseases.

2. Many severe diseases result from a hereditary disposition.

3. Just as when two straight lines diverge from each other by an interval which, scarcely perceptible when the lines are close together, becomes a vast difference if the lines are extended into infinity, so small deviations from the natural state, in the uterus, become notably increased when the infant grows up.

4. Any climate and any age, and each sex, has its special diseases.

5. The positions of the sun and the moon, their location and movement, exert great power over our bodies; thus, in the solstices and equinoxes a noteworthy change takes place in our body.

6. The seasons of the year may be the causes of various diseases; hence in spring those diseases are more frequent which involve many humours, and in autumn those which result from corruption.

7. The nature of the spirits (which direct our machine and bring about health) depend in very great part on the blood. Air, food, drink, and age induce variations in the composition of the blood.

8. The air can variously affect the humours of our body and the solid parts, through moisture, dryness, heat and cold; and, through the variations of the effluvia, even has great power to change the texture and proportion of the blood.

9. In almost any region and place certain diseases are familiar because of the differing constitution of the air.

10. Through uneven quality and sudden change of the air the blood is variously affected, and our machine very greatly disturbed in its operations.

[. . .]

Chapter 5: Of diseases arising from uneven and impeded circulation of the blood

1. The most important circumstance of life and health lies in the circulation of the blood. Here, therefore, should be sought the origin of many diseases.

2. From uneven and impeded circulation of the blood there

arises syncope, which is the extinction of vital actions when the movement of the heart and the arteries stops.

3. The motion of the heart is the primary cause and basis of the circulation of the blood. When that motion stops, the circulation ceases and at the same time are abolished all the actions that proceed from life.

4. For the motion of the heart it is not enough to have an influx of animal spirits, but we also require an internal movement of the blood and a suitable mixture of blood. If that inflow of spirits ceases and the internal movement and the mixture of the blood are done away with, the motion of the heart is abolished.

[. . .]

20. When the blood collects more abundantly in the very small vessels, it stagnates there and produces a troublesome sense of pain and heat, until, gradually corrupted, it changes into pus or sanies; the first of these changes is called inflammation or phlegmon, the latter, abscess or aposteme.

21. For the most part the cause of inflammation is an irregular destructive salt having an angular configuration, which in a troublesome fashion stimulates the nerve fibres and membranes, contracts them spasmodically, narrows the capillary veins, and thus hinders the circulation of the blood.

Herman Boerhaave

In the first half of the eighteenth century Herman Boerhaave was probably Europe's greatest physician. Born in 1668, he received his medical degree in 1693, taught and practised in Leiden, and died in 1738. While he made no great discoveries, nor propounded any revolutionary doctrines, he was an outstanding clinician and teacher and a prominent chemist. Yet these facts alone do not explain his great influence.

Boerhaave represented a stabilizing force in a world which was undergoing great intellectual turmoil as well as social, political and economic commotion. In the latter seventeenth century the Galenic tradition was crumbling, and amid the resulting confusion the rival doctrines of the iatrophysicists and iatrochemists competed with those of quacks and empirics. Rationalism and empiricism each had their proponents. The authority of Aristotle was losing ground to the mechanical and chemical philosophies. A 'modern' trend was struggling with an entrenched establishment. Pointing up the conflict was the great quarrel between the ancients and the moderns, wherein the traditional learning fought a losing fight. The intellectual climate suffered from great unrest.

In the seventeenth century new discoveries opened new perspectives in medicine and biology. The concept of the circulation, the whole new world which the microscope disclosed, the revelations of the telescope, the advances in physics and chemistry, anatomy and physiology, produced a tremendous influx of new facts with which the old conceptual schema was incapable of dealing. The data of microscopy and of chemistry provided material which seemed basic to medical science, and which had to be taken account of. New facts produced new theories. We have seen that Friederich Hoffmann tried to integrate some of the new information into a new system, but he did so in a relatively crude form. Boerhaave's great merit was the creation of a system that synthesized many different strands and threads into a complete fabric, a system which satisfied the needs of the times and gained widespread acceptance. He summarized the knowledge of the time and integrated it into a well-rounded whole where every part had its relationship to every other part and all data could find suitable explanation from the initial premises.

Boerhaave, in 1708, published his *Institutes* which went through several editions in many languages. The actual text consists of short concentrated paragraphs comparable to lecture headings, and needing expansion. After Boerhaave's death his pupil Haller provided annotations to the original text, annotations which, drawn from notes, expand the thought and provide invaluable exposition. The standard English edition of Boerhaave's *Institutes* derives from the Haller edition. Our quotations are taken from the introductory section, in which Boerhaave discussed methodology.

In the eighteenth century the most disreputable word to a physician was 'hypothesis', a word which implied speculation and imagination without adequate logical or empirical foundation. Sound medicine depended on two elements – observation, i.e., knowledge gained through the senses; and reasoning, i.e., knowledge gained through logical inference. Sound inference permitted 'just' conclusions – that is, those which were logical, reliable, valid. The systematist realized that the corporeal eye had its limitation and could see only a limited distance into the phenomena of nature. To understand nature the corporeal eye must be supplemented by the eye of reason, which could penetrate more deeply.

In the selections given here Boerhaave discussed some points of methodology. As a rationalist and systematist, he believed firmly that his own observations and his inferences were 'just' while those of his predecessors were merely 'hypotheses'. Grounding his doctrines primarily on the mechanical philosophy, he explained the various phenomena of health and disease through concepts which had a minimal basis of experience and a great deal of theoretical elaboration. In these brief excerpts we are not able to give details of Boerhaave's system, which would illustrate its hypothetical character. A detailed exposition I have given elsewhere.

9 Academical Lectures on the Theory of Physic (1741)

Excerpts from *Dr Boerhaave's Academical Lectures on the Theory of Physic*, vol. 1, W. Innys, 1751, pp. 51–76. [The annotations and footnotes are renumbered.]

Of the parts and principles[1] of physic

20. Physic has been loaded with many *useless*[2] and *fallacious*[3] *hypotheses*; to *expel*[4] *which*, we are to consider that the whole design of the art is to keep off and remove pain, sickness and death, and therefore, to preserve present and restore lost health; so that every thing necessary to be known by a physician, is reducible to one of these two heads.

21. The *object* therefore of physic in the human body, is life, health, disease, and death, with the causes from whence they

1. By *Principles* we here understand, not the constituent parts or elements of bodies, but the means of demonstration, or truths; not depending upon others, but by which others are to be established.

2. Among the useless hypotheses, we may reckon that of the Pythagoreans, explaining the nature of bodies by numbers; the subtile matter of the *Cartesians*; a subtile and rambling ether; the *Fuga Vacui*, etc. But the ingenuity of mankind has been generally unwilling to take up with such principles as are the most obvious to our senses, and useful to our interest; they think we cannot understand nutrition, unless we are first acquainted with the nature of wheat, nor can we understand the nature of that, unless we are acquainted with the nature of the constituent principles. But their search does even not terminate in the constituent principles or elements, but they must endeavour to find out by conjecture in what manner the universal matter of all things does by a substantial form put on the texture and disposition of wheat. But if these things were possible to be known, as they certainly are not, they would have no manner of use with regard to the affairs of human life.

3. Such is the nature of fallacious hypotheses, that when the principles which are laid down for the basis are only imaginary, the whole train of consequences which are thence deduced, must be evidently false, and amount to nothing.[. . .]

4. Every thing which does not conduce to the preservation of health, and to the cure of diseases, may be purposely omitted in physic, notwithstanding they may be both true and curious: because a physician may perform his office without their assistance.

arise, and the means by which they are to be regulated, restored, or prevented.

22. Physic is therefore the *science* or knowledge of those things, by whose application and effects health may be preserved when present, and restored when lost, by the cure of diseases.

23. Therefore the necessity, *usefulness* and *dignity* of physic, are hence sufficiently apparent.

24. There are two methods which may be relied upon as certain for the attainment of our profession, which may be esteemed its solid foundations; the first is an accurate *observation*[5] of all the appearances offered to our senses in the human body, whether in *health*,[6] *diseases*,[7] *dying*,[8] or already *dead*;[9] whether they proceed from internal causes residing in the animal, or from the action of external bodies, accidents, or the art itself. The second is a strict consideration and discovery of the several latent causes, concealed from our naked *senses*[10] in human bodies, by a just

5. Observation here is the attention of the mind to such changes as happen in human bodies, all which changes proceed from motion, which motion is produced originally in the body, as a machine; some of these changes are obvious to the senses, others are not so.[. . .]

6. The state of the pulse, and respiration, the colour, heat, tension, and moisture of the skin, the brightness of the eyes, etc. as they appear in healthy bodies, in order to distinguish the morbid changes in the same appearances; from a due consideration of all these signs, may be deduced an estimate of the danger, or the probability of recovery, and state of the powers of life, or of the disease; all which were largely considered by the ancients, but have undeservedly been treated with much neglect in the present age.

7. By enquiring into all the present circumstances of the patient's case, and by asking him and his attendants after every thing, which will not fall under his cognizance without.

8. [. . .] We indeed say a man is dying when the disease prevails and tends to death; thus in a phrenitis, which will prove fatal on the fourth day, the patient begins to die in the middle of the third day, and the whole system of the body, especially the brain, is gradually destroyed.

9. To search out by practical anatomy the latent causes of diseases, of which we are often so greatly ignorant, and to remark all the changes which have been made by death throughout the whole body, and all its viscera. [. . .]

10. An instance of this we have in the *sanctorian* perspiration, a discovery of the utmost consequence in physic, which that author observed in his own person, and has done more service to physic than all the subtle imaginary schemes and interpretations of Galen, which were made during the whole thirteenth century. [. . .] We ought to make it our chief study to collect all the observations and experiments we possibly can, and dispose them under their proper heads; but an experiment or fact is with regard to the thing

reasoning[11]; which is really necessary, to prevent future ill accidents, and secure the good events. Physic thus established upon judgment and observation, can be only attained by a just reasoning from the several facts, which have before been thoroughly considered[12] in every respect; from comparing those reasonings with nature or experience, and with each other; and from diligently remarking which of them appear agreeable or disagreeable to truth; that from the whole we may be enabled to draw just conclusions in regard to present and future events; which conclusions may then be relied upon[13] with certainty as matter of fact.

25. In order to discover truth in this manner by observation and reason, it is requisite we should fix on some principles whose certainty and effects are *demonstrable*[14] to our senses, which may

itself, an appearance obvious to the senses of the enquirer; our mind adds nothing to the appearance, but barely the perception of it.

11. We are said to reason when we compare the ideas we have before experienced with each other, that we may be distinctly informed of every property appertaining to each idea, and thence form a judgment of the agreement or difference between each; nor is there any thing more required to knowledge, than this comparison distinctly and patiently prosecuted. But the physician above all stands in need of just reasoning, to assist him in the discovery in many things of the human body, particularly the great class of diseases which lie concealed from the observation of naked sense; God has also given reasonable faculties to our minds to make new discoveries of truth and invention; we cannot expect such discoveries from careless observation, and accidental experiment, but from those which are designedly made with a strict attention of mind, to convert them to some use. Observation or experience alone will not make a physician; for any two diseases are never so much alike, but a small degree of reasoning may distinguish the difference.

12. All the observations which we have made upon any head ought to be committed to paper, examined with the strictest attention, and applied to the present circumstances of our patient's cafe, that by considering every particular, we may by a slow and solid judgment determine the latent causes of diseases. [. . .]

13. If physicians were to unite their endeavours, and form a society for the collecting of every thing true and useful from the writings we now possess, and afterwards digest them into aphorisms under proper heads, it must certainly form a system of physic capable of solving any difficulty in the art with as equal certainty as the problems in any other science.

14. Demonstration is an evident proof of some dubious proposition, so that no body who admits the general principles, can deny their assent; these are purest in the mathematics, though there are many demonstrations no

serve to explain the phenomena[15] of natural bodies, and account for the accidents that arise in them; such only are those which are purely material in the human body, with *mechanical*[16] and physical experiments; for we are not sensible of any other way of attaining to a true knowledge of the universal and particular affections of bodies.

26. But as there are in the human body many other appearances[17] not intelligible upon those principles, they therefore are not to be demonstrated and explained by such principles. [. . .]

27. We are to consider, (i) that man is composed of a *body*[18] and *mind*,[19] *united*[20] to each other; (ii) that the *nature*[21] of these are

less evident in physic, especially those which are taken from anatomy. But there is no necessity for the principles of any art to be proved in that art, it is sufficient if their certainty is by any means demonstrated in other arts.

15. These ought to be first adjusted with distinction, clearness and certainty; with distinction, which points out one being from any other; [. . .] with clearness, which consists of simple motions or ideas easily conceived by any man in his senses, as that two and two joined make four; with certainty, which cannot be denied by any reasonable person, or which must always appear true upon examination.

16. The universal laws of nature, or affections of all bodies, depend on mechanical and physical principles, upon which alone their actions are explicable; the same laws are also true in the human body, for its matter appears to be universally the same with that of all other bodies; so that what may be said to be true of all bodies, may be also affirmed true in our own. Thus, if one should affirm, that by the friction of two bodies would arise heat, the same will also be true upon the friction of solid parts in the human body. [. . .]

17. Such as memory, understanding, reason and the knowledge of past and future appearances; which are peculiar to the mind, a being without figure or extension, and conscious of pleasure and pain.

18. By the body we understand that part of us which is extended in three dimensions, has a form and is fitted for motion or rest, etc.

19. By the mind we understand that being which thinks, and perceives itself thinking, and the thing thought of.

20. The union of the body and mind is such, that the mind cannot resist forming to itself the ideas of pleasure and pain, when the body is in a particular manner affected; nor can the healthy body refuse to obey the action of the mind under particular circumstances.

21. By the nature of the body or mind, we understand everything which we are satisfied belong to each. The essential nature of the mind is to be conscious, or to think; but to think of this and that particular thing, is accidental to it. The essential nature of the body is extension and resistance. These attributes have nothing in common to each other. [. . .]

very different, and that therefore, (iii) each has a *life*,[22] *actions*[23] and affections differing from the other; yet (iv) that there is such a reciprocal connection and consent between the particular thoughts and affections of the mind and the body, that a change in one always produces a change in the other, and the reverse; also, (v) that the mind performs some actions by mere thought, without any effect upon the body; and that it has other thoughts, which arise barely from some change in the condition of the body; on the other hand also, (vi) that there are some actions performed by the body without the attention, knowledge or desire of the mind, which is neither concerned therein as the cause or effect of those actions; that there are also some ideas formed in the mind of a person in health by its past actions; and lastly, that there are other ideas compounded both of the past and present. That, (vii) whatever we observe to arise from thought in the human body, is to be only ascribed to the mind as the cause. But, (viii) that every appearance which has solidity, figure or motion, is to be ascribed to the body and its motion for a principle, and ought to be demonstrated and explained by their properties. That, (ix) we cannot understand or explain the manner in which the body and mind reciprocally act upon each other from any consideration of their separate nature; we can only (x) remark by observation their effects upon each other, without

---

22. The life of the body is: (i) to generate motion under particular circumstances, as the loadstone approaches to iron. (ii) For its constituent parts to attract each other, from whence proceeds that resistance to the force of external bodies, or *vis inertia*. (iii) To gravitate, or tend towards the centre of its planet. And then (iv) comes the affections proper to particular bodies. The life of the mind is: (i) to perceive the appearances of all external objects, by the changes they make in the organs of sensation. (ii) To judge or compare the nature of two ideas with each other, and then to deduce some consequence, as that they are of the same kind, or different; as we conclude from our notions of a circle and triangle, that a triangle is not a circle. (iii) To will anything. In a word, the life of the mind is, to be conscious. These are all the functions of the mind; for past actions are uncertain, and they may be all referred to the single act of its consciousness.

23. The action of the body is to communicate motion to other bodies; the passion of it is to receive some change in itself from another body or a mind. The action of the mind is volition, which every body is acquainted with, but no one can explain. The passions of the mind are the changes it receives from external objects by the senses. [. . .]

explaining them; and when any difficulty or appearance has been traced so far, that it only remains to explain the manner of their reciprocal action, we are to suppose such account *satisfactory*,[24] both because it may be sufficient for all the purposes of the physician, and as it is impossible for him to search any further.

28. We may also affirm, that the *primary physical causes*,[25] in what manner, and the ultimate *metaphysical causes*,[26] for what end, the soft general appearances are in a determinate manner affected, are neither possible, useful, or necessary to be investigated by a physician; such as the origin of primitive and *feminal forms*, of *motion*, the *elements*, etc.

29. But a physician may, and ought to furnish himself with

24. [. . .] We call an explanation of a thing the demonstration of agreement or relation between its own properties and the same in another; but this is here not only impossible, but also quite useless to a physician; for the great business of a physician is to be acquainted with the means of restoring lost health, and no cure can be effected by him, but through some change made in the human body by the application of others; therefore this search after the connection between the body and mind not appertaining to a physician, is to be rejected, among those (20) which are useless to the art. The physician, who cures diseases of the body, is not solicitous about those of the mind; for when the first is set to rights, the latter will quickly return to its office. Thus when the eye is blinded with a cataract, the mind cannot perceive sensible objects by it, the aid of physic is therefore called in to couch the cataract, or depress the opaque crystalline *lens*; after which the rays of light finding a free admission to the *retina*, the mind will be sensible of visible objects by it; and thus the business of physic will be done without the assistance of optics. When a person is in a *delirium*, or swoon, the physician cannot recall the mind, which has no relation to his business; but by applying vinegar, or other volatiles to the nose, he can restore the sick machine to its former motions, and then the mind will also exhibit its former actions, and this full as well as if he understood the manner of connection between the actions of the body and those of the conscious mind.

25. *Primary causes* are those productive of secondary ones; but we always meet with God in our search after these, and this puts a stop to our further knowledge; for God is an infinite being, and if we compare the whole universe with him, it will be found almost nothing. In our search after *physical causes*, we should not be over solicitous to determine everything in which experiment will not assist us; for we never can be certain of the truth of such discoveries, and if we were, it would be of little or no use to mankind. [. . .] We ought therefore to rest upon experiment, and lay aside useless attempts to explain the most general laws and principles observed in nature. [. . .]

26. By metaphysical causes, are meant those general attributes of beings which are abstractedly essential to them as beings. [. . .]

and reason from, such things as are demonstrated to be true in *anatomy*,[27] *chemistry*[28] and *mechanics*,[29] with natural and experimental *philosophy*, provided he confines his reasoning within the bounds of truth and simple experiment (25).

30. It is necessary for the physician, in furnishing himself with these principles and experiments, to begin first with such as are most simple, certain and easy to be understood; after which he may proceed to those which are more compounded, and so by degrees to the most complex, obscure, and difficult.

31. He that would learn by experiments, ought to proceed from particulars to generals; but the method of instructing academically, proceeds from generals to particulars; [. . .].

27. He that desires to learn truth, should teach himself by facts and experiments; by which means he will know more in a year; than by abstract reasoning in an age. Proper experiments have always truth to defend them; also reasoning joined with mathematical evidence, and founded upon experiment, will hold equally true ; but should it be true, without those supports it must be altogether useless. Nature distributes the faculty of reason to all men equally alike, but he will excel in reasoning who has made the best use of experiments, having considered the structure, situation, figure, size and other peculiarities obvious to our senses in the several parts of the human body.

28. Chemistry acquaints us with those changes which arise in bodies from mixture, and the application of them to fire. Suppose one substance of a particular kind to be mixed with another, and applied to a determinate degree of fire, the consequence will be a production of new appearances, which is the business of the chemist to remark; nor does ever chemistry deceive us, if it proceeds no farther than real experiments, and their effects; upon the addition of the best oil of cloves to rectified oil of vitriol, they run into a violent commotion, and exhale clouds as thick as pitch, which quickly turn into flames.

29. Mechanics teach us to apply the general laws of motion to all kinds of bodies. Every body is extended, resists motion, is moveable, capable of form, etc. The effects of all these general qualities, and the moving powers thence arising, are applicable to every particular body; nor can we be deceived therein, if the body to which they are applied be distinctly and carefully considered in all those respects. Mechanics therefore supposes a previous knowledge of the structure of all the parts in the human body, to which we would apply mechanical laws; and in this sense physic is no more than the knowledge of such things as are transacted in the human body.

[. . .]

William Cullen

William Cullen, born in 1710 in Scotland, was the successor of Boerhaave so far as the English-speaking countries were concerned. Primarily a clinician, he was well versed in chemistry, even though he did not make any significant contributions to this science. His great claim to fame was his ability as a teacher and a practitioner, and his gift for systematizing and clarifying the knowledge of the time. In the rationalist tradition he tried to create an over-arching system that would account for all the data and would explain them in a logical and satisfying manner. One of his great contributions was the classification of diseases, a nosology which, as a work of classification, illustrates well the rationalistic tendencies of the time.

His most influential work, the *First Lines of the Practice of Physic*, went through many editions. Clinically orientated, it avoided the abstract and theoretical dogmatism and the concern with first principles that we note in Hoffmann, but nevertheless illustrates well the lack of critical acumen that permeated eighteenth-century rationalism. In his preface he indicated some of the ideals that he tried to follow, and he paid lip service to the need for solid and empirical evidence. He genuinely believed that he himself avoided 'hypotheses', and that he was relying on facts and cautious induction therefrom. However, as we see in the excerpts that discuss the causes and mechanisms of some specific diseases, he indulged in unsupported statements and uncritical hypotheses.

Cullen died in 1790. He was a great clinician and teacher, who helped to make Edinburgh the leading medical school of the latter part of the eighteenth century and who exerted great influence on medicine in America as well as in Great Britain. But he stands in rather sharp contrast to the empirical trend which was gathering strength. For representatives of this trend we can turn to James Lind and John Hunter.

10 First Lines of the Practice of Physic (1786)

Excerpts from W. Cullen, *First Lines of the Practice of Physic*, vol. 1, C. Elliot: Edinburgh; T. Cadell: London, 1786, pp. xiii–lvi, 64–9, 86–103.

Preface

[. . .] I apprehend that, in every branch of science with respect to which new facts are daily acquired, and these consequently giving occasion to new reflections, which correct the principles formerly adopted, it is necessary, from time to time, to reform and renew the whole system, with all the additions and amendments which it has received and is then capable of. That at present this is requisite with regard to the science of medicine, will, I believe, readily occur to every person who at all thinks for himself, and is acquainted with the systems which have hitherto prevailed. [. . .]

I have endeavoured to collect the facts relative to the diseases of the human body, as fully as the nature of the work and the bounds necessarily prescribed to it would admit. But I have not been satisfied with giving the facts, without endeavouring to apply them to the investigation of proximate causes, and upon these to establish a more scientific and decided method of cure. In aiming at this, I flatter myself that I have avoided hypothesis, and what have been called *theories*. I have, indeed, endeavoured to establish many general doctrines, both physiological and pathological; but I trust that these are only a generalization of facts, or conclusions from a cautious and full induction: and if any one shall refuse to admit, or directly shall oppose, my general doctrines, he must do it by showing that I have been deficient or mistaken in assuming and applying facts. I have, myself, been jealous of my being sometimes imperfect in these respects; but I have generally endeavoured to obviate the consequences of this, by proving, that the proximate causes which I have assigned, are true in fact, as well as deductions from any reasoning that I may seem to have employed. Further, to obviate any dangerous fallacy in proposing a method of cure, I have always been anxious to suggest that which, to the best of my judgement, appeared to be the method approved of by experience, as much as it was the consequence of system.

Upon this general plan I have endeavoured to form a system of physic that should comprehend the whole of the facts relating to the science, and that will, I hope, collect and arrange them in better order than has been done before, as well as point out in particular those which are still wanting to establish general principles. This which I have attempted, may, like other systems, hereafter suffer a change; but I am confident that we are at present in a better train of investigation than physicians were in before the time of Dr Hoffmann.

Of pyrexiae, or febrile diseases

6. Pyrexiae, or febrile diseases, are distinguished by the following appearances. After beginning with some degree of cold shivering, they show some increase of heat, and an increased frequency of pulse, with the interruption and disorder of several functions, particularly some diminution of strength in the animal functions.

7. Of these Pyrexiae I have formed a class, and have subdivided it into the five orders of *fevers*, *inflammations*, *eruptions*, *haemorrhages*, and *fluxes*.

Of fevers

Of the phenomena of fevers. 8. Those diseases are more strictly called *fevers*, which have the general symptoms of pyrexia, without having along with them any topical affection that is essential and primary, such as the other orders of the pyrexiæ always have.

9. Fevers, as differing in the number and variety of their symptoms, have been very properly considered as of distinct genera and species. But we suppose, that there are certain circumstances in common to all the diseases comprehended under this order, which are therefore those essentially necessary to, and properly constituting the nature of fever. It is our business especially, and in the first place, to investigate these; and I expect to find them as they occur in the paroxysm, or fit, of an intermittent fever, as this is most commonly formed.

10. The phenomena to be observed in such a paroxysm are the following. The person is affected, first, with a languor or sense

of debility, a sluggishness in motion, and some uneasiness in exerting it, with frequent yawning and stretching. At the same time, the face and extremities become pale; the features shrink; the bulk of every external part is diminished; and the skin, over the whole body, appears constricted, as if cold had been applied to it. At the coming on of these symptoms, some coldness of the extremities, though little taken notice of by the patient, may be perceived by another person. At length, the patient himself feels a sensation of cold, commonly first in his back, but, from thence, passing over the whole body; and now his skin feels warm to another person. The patient's sense of cold increasing, produces a tremor in all his limbs, with frequent successions or rigors of the trunk of the body. When this sense of cold, and its effects, have continued for some time, they become less violent, and are alternated with warm flushings. By degrees, the cold goes off entirely; and a heat, greater than natural, prevails, and continues over the whole body. With this heat, the colour of the skin returns, and a preternatural redness appears, especially in the face. Whilst the heat and redness come on, the skin is relaxed and smoothed, but, for some time, continues dry. The features of the face, and other parts of the body, recover their usual size, and become even more turgid. When the heat, redness, and turgescence have increased and continued for some time, a moisture appears upon the forehead, and by degrees becomes a sweat, which gradually extends downwards over the whole body. As this sweat continues to flow, the heat of the body abates; the sweat, after continuing some time, gradually ceases; the body returns to its usual temperature; and most of the functions are restored to their ordinary state.

11. This series of appearances gives occasion to divide the paroxysm into three different stages; which are called the *cold*, the *hot*, and the *sweating stages* or *fits*.

[. . .]

Of the proximate cause of fever. 33. The proximate cause of fever seems hitherto to have eluded the research of physicians; and I shall not pretend to ascertain it in a manner that may remove every difficulty; but I shall endeavour to make an approach towards it, and such as, I hope, may be of use in conducting the practice in this disease: while at the same time I hope to avoid several errors which have formerly prevailed on this subject.

34. As the hot stage of fever is so constantly preceded by a cold stage, we presume that the latter is the cause of the former; and, therefore, that the cause of the cold stage is the cause of all that follows in the course of the paroxysm.

35. To discover the cause of the cold stage of fevers, we may observe, that it is always preceded by strong marks of a general debility prevailing in the system. The smallness and weakness of the pulse, the paleness and coldness of the extreme parts, with the shrinking of the whole body, sufficiently show that the action of the heart and larger arteries is, for the time, extremely weakened. Together with this, the languor, inactivity, and debility of the animal motions, the imperfect sensations, the feeling of cold, while the body is truly warm, and some other symptoms, all show that the energy of the brain is, on this occasion, greatly weakened; and I presume, that, as the weakness of the action of the heart can hardly be imputed to any other cause, this weakness also is a proof of the diminished energy of the brain.

36. I shall hereafter endeavour to show, that the most noted of the remote causes of fever, as contagion, miasmata, cold and fear, are of a sedative nature; and therefore render it probable that a debility is induced. Likewise, when the paroxysms of a fever have ceased to be repeated, they may again be renewed, and are most commonly renewed by the application of debilitating powers. And, further, the debility which subsists in the animal motions and other functions through the whole of fever, renders it pretty certain that sedative or debilitating powers have been applied to the body.

37. It is therefore evident, that there are three states which always take place in fever; a state of debility, a state of cold, and a state of heat; and as these three states regularly and constantly succeed each other in the order we have mentioned them, it is presumed that they are in the series of cause and effect with respect to one another. This we hold as a matter of fact, even although we should not be able to explain in what manner or by what mechanical means these states severally produce each other.

38. How the state of debility produces some of the symptoms of the cold stage, may perhaps be readily explained; but how it pro-

duces all of them, I cannot explain otherwise than by referring the matter to a general law of the animal-economy, whereby it happens, that powers which have a tendency to hurt and destroy the system, often excite such motions as are suited to obviate the effects of the noxious power. This is the *vis medicatrix naturae*, so famous in the schools of physic; and it seems probable, that many of the motions excited in fever are the effects of this power.

39. That the increased action of the heart and arteries, which takes place in the hot stage of fevers, is to be considered as an effort of the *vis medicatrix naturae*, has been long a common opinion among physicians; and I am disposed to assert, that some part of the cold stage may be imputed to the same power. [. . .]

40. It is to be particularly observed, that, during the cold stage of fever, there seems to be a spasm induced everywhere on the extremities of the arteries, and more especially of those upon the surface of the body. This appears from the suppression of all excretions, and from the shrinking of the external parts: and although this may perhaps be imputed, in part, to the weaker action of the heart in propelling the blood into the extreme vessels; yet, as these symptoms often continue after the action of the heart is restored, there is reason to believe, that a spasmodic constriction has taken place; that it subsists for some time, and supports the hot stage; for this stage ceases with the flowing of the sweat, and the return of other excretions, which are marks of the relaxation of vessels formerly constricted.

41. The idea of fever, then, may be, that a spasm of the extreme vessels, however induced, proves an irritation to the heart and arteries; and that this continues till the spasm is relaxed or overcome. There are many appearances which support this opinion; and there is little doubt that a spasm does take place, which proves an irritation to the heart, and therefore may be considered as a principal part in the proximate cause of fever. It will still, however, remain a question, what is the cause of this spasm; whether it be directly produced by the remote causes of fever, or it it be only a part of the operation of the *vis medicatrix naturae*.

42. I am disposed to be of the latter opinion. [. . .]

43. It is therefore presumed, that such a cold fit and spasm at the beginning of fever, is a part of the operation of the *vis medicatrix*;

but, at the same time, it seems to me probable, that, during the whole course of the fever, there is an atony subsisting in the extreme vessels, and that the relaxation of the spasm requires the restoring of the tone and action of these.

44. This it may be difficult to explain; but I think it may be ascertained as a fact, by the consideration of the symptoms which take place with respect to the functions of the stomach in fevers, such as the anorexia, nausea, and vomiting.

From many circumstances it is sufficiently certain that there is a consent between the stomach and surface of the body; and in all cases of the consent of distant parts, it is presumed to be by the connection of the nervous system, and that the consent which appears is between the sentient and moving fibres of the one part with those of the other; is such, that a certain condition prevailing in the one part occasions a similar condition in the other.

In the case of the stomach and surface of the body, the consent particularly appears by the connection which is observed between the state of the perspiration and the state of the appetite in healthy persons; and if it may be presumed that the appetite depends upon the state of tone in the muscular fibres of the stomach, it will follow, that the connection of appetite and perspiration depends upon a consent between the muscular fibres of the stomach and the muscular fibres of the extreme vessels, or of the organ of perspiration, on the surface of the body.

It is further in proof of the connection between the appetite and perspiration, and at the same time of the circumstances on which it depends, that cold applied to the surface of the body, when it does not stop perspiration, but proves a stimulus to it, is always a powerful means of exciting appetite.

Having thus established the connection or consent mentioned, we argue that as the symptoms of anorexia, nausea and vomiting, in many cases, manifestly depend upon a state of debility or loss of tone in the muscular fibres of the stomach, so it may be presumed, that these symptoms, in the beginning of fever, depend upon an atony communicated to the muscular fibres of the stomach from the muscular fibres of the extreme vessels on the surface of the body.

[. . .]

From the whole we have now said on this subject, I think it is sufficiently probable that the symptoms of anorexia, nausea and vomiting, depend upon, and are a proof of, an atony subsisting in the extreme vessels on the surface of the body; and that this atony therefore, now ascertained as a matter of fact, may be considered as a principal circumstance in the proximate cause of fever.

45. This atony we suppose to depend upon a diminution of the energy of the brain; and that this diminution takes place in fevers, we conclude not only from the debility prevailing in so many of the functions of the body, mentioned above, but particularly from symptoms which are peculiar to the brain itself. Delirium is a frequent symptom of fever: and as from the physiology and pathology we learn that this symptom commonly depends upon some inequality in the excitement of the brain or intellectual organ; we hence conclude, that, in fever, it denotes some diminution in the energy of the brain. [. . .]

46. Upon the whole, our doctrine of fever is explicitly this. The remote causes are certain sedative powers applied to the nervous system, which diminishing the energy of the brain, thereby produce a debility in the whole of the functions, and particularly in the action of the extreme vessels. Such, however, is, at the same time, the nature of the animal economy, that this debility proves an indirect stimulus to the sanguiferous system; whence, by the intervention of the cold stage, and spasm connected with it, the action of the heart and larger arteries is increased, and continues so till it has had the effect of restoring the energy of the brain, of extending this energy to the extreme vessels, of restoring therefore their action, and thereby especially overcoming the spasm affecting them; upon the removing of which, the excretion of sweat, and other marks of the relaxation of excretories, take place.

James Lind

James Lind achieved fame and success the hard way. Born in Edinburgh in 1716, he entered medicine by what we may call the 'low road'. At the age of fifteen he was apprenticed to a surgeon. At the age of twenty-three he joined the British navy, in which he served for nine years. Only after he left the navy, in 1748, did he get his MD degree from the University of Edinburgh. Then he settled down to practice. Most of his later life he served as physician to a naval hospital near Portsmouth and he died in 1794.

Lind's *Treatise on Scurvy*, published in 1753, is one of the finest clinical studies ever written. It is excellent clinical research, combining careful observation of disease, penetrating analysis of possible factors involved, precise experimentation, cautious drawing of conclusion. Lind was not a 'trained' scientist. He did not possess special technical knowledge in basic disciplines such as chemistry or physiology, but he did observe the patient, thought about the patient and devised his experiments about the patient. At no time did he lose sight of the patient-as-a-whole.

At the very beginning of the selection here quoted, we see a contrast between clinical observation and laboratory research. Lind described the attempts of a chemist to find a suitable remedy for scurvy. The chemist worked in his laboratory and then sent the medicines overseas to be tested. They all proved ineffectual and the efforts served as a pointed commentary on the dangers of separating 'laboratory' investigation from clinical investigation.

But even more important than the actual concern with the bedside is the clear thinking that Lind exhibited – *scientific method* at its best. He worked with only a few patients, but they were carefully 'controlled', as carefully as the circumstances would permit. His experimental work climaxed a long period of observation and reflection, and wide acquaintance with the efforts of others.

Interestingly enough, the cogency of Lind's demonstration did not particularly impress his contemporaries, and his recommendations did not gain wide acceptance for many years. Scientific acumen can become effective only in a favourable environment, and in the mid-eighteenth century that environment was not yet ready.

11 A Treatise on the Scurvy (1753)

Excerpts from J. Lind, 'A Treatise on the Scurvy' in C. P. Stewart and
D. Guthrie (eds.), *Lind's Treatise on Scurvy*, Edinburgh University Press,
1953, pp. 139–53.

Of the prevention of scurvy

[. . .]

A German who had acquired a considerable fortune in East
Indies, by being Dutch Governor of Sumatra, was so affected
with pity and humanity for the many afflicted sailors he had
observed in this malady, that, imagining the art of chemistry,
which at that time made a great noise in the world, might probably furnish some remedy for their relief, he erected and endowed a perpetual professorship of that science at Leipzig. He
nominated his countryman Dr Michael, a very great chemist,
who was the first university professor of chemistry in Europe;
and remitted him a considerable sum of money, in order to bear
the expence of his experiments, with the promise of a much
greater, in case he succeeded in the discovery of a remedy for
prevention of the scurvy at sea. The doctor spent an incredible
deal of time and labour in preparing the most elaborated chemical
medicines. Volatile and fixed salts, spirits of all sorts, essences,
elixirs, electuaries, etc. were yearly sent over to the East Indies;
[. . .]. But all proved ineffectual.

Bontekoe recommended to the Dutch sailors an acrid alkaline
spirit; Glauber and Boerhaave, a strong mineral acid, viz. *sp.
salis*. The Royal Navy of Great Britain has been supplied, at a
considerable expence to the government, by the advice of an
eminent physician, with a large quantity of elixir of vitriol; which
is the strong mineral acid of vitriol combined with aromatics.
Wine-vinegar was likewise prescribed upon this occasion by the
college of physicians at London [. . .]. Vinegar has been indeed
much used in the fleet at all times. Many ships, especially those
fitted out at Plymouth, carried with them cider for this purpose,
upon the recommendation of the learned Dr Huxham. The
latest proposal to the Lords of the Admiralty was a magazine of
dried spinach prepared in the manner of hay. This was to be

moistened and boiled in their food. To which it was objected by a very ingenious physician, that no moisture whatever could restore the natural juices of the plant lost by evaporation, and, as he imagined, altered by a fermentation which they underwent in drying.

Moreover, all the remedies which could be used in the circumstances of sailors, that at any time have been proposed for the many various diseases going under the name of a scurvy at land, have likewise been tried to prevent and cure this disease at sea. [. . .]

Experience has abundantly shown, that they have not been sufficient to prevent this disease, much less to cure it. And the same may be said of many others. The consequence of which is, the world has now almost despaired of finding out a method of preventing this dreadful evil at sea; and it is become the received opinion, that it is altogether impossible there, either to prevent or cure it. But it is surprising, that this ill-grounded belief, so fatal in its consequences, should have gained credit, when we see people recovering from this disease every day, (even in the most deplorable condition, and in its last stages), in a short time, when proper helps are administered. [. . .]

What I propose is, first, to relate the effects of several medicines tried at sea in this disease, on purpose to discover what might promise the most certain protection against it upon that element. [. . .]

The following are the experiments.

On 20 May 1747, I took twelve patients in the scurvy, on board the *Salisbury* at sea. Their cases were as similar as I could have them. They all in general had putrid gums, the spots and lassitude, with weakness of their knees. They lay together in one place, being a proper apartment for the sick in the fore-hold; and had one diet common to all, viz. water-gruel sweetened with sugar in the morning; fresh mutton-broth often times for dinner; at other times puddings, boiled biscuit with sugar, etc.; and for supper, barley and raisins, rice and currants, sago and wine, or the like. Two of these were ordered each a quart of cider a day. Two others took twenty-five gutts [drops] of elixir vitriol three times a day, upon an empty stomach; using a gargle strongly acidulated with it for their mouths. Two others took two spoonfuls of vinegar three times a day, upon an empty stomach; having their gruels and their other food well acidulated with it, as also the gargle for their mouth. Two of the worst patients, with the tendons in the ham rigid, (a symptom none of the rest had), were put under a course of sea-water. Of this they drank half a pint every day, and sometimes more or less as it operated, by way of gentle physic. Two others had each two oranges and one lemon given them every day. These they eat with greediness, at different times, upon an empty stomach. They continued but six days under this course, having consumed the quantity that could be spared. The two remaining patients, took the bigness of a nutmeg three times a day, of an electuary recommended by an hospital surgeon, made of garlic, mustard-seed, *rad. raphan.* balsam of Peru and gum myrrh; using for common drink, barley-water well acidulated with tamarinds; by a decoction of which, with the addition of *cremor tartar*, they were gently purged three of four times during the course.

The consequence was, that the most sudden and visible good effects were perceived from the use of the oranges and lemons; one of those who had taken them, being at the end of six days fit for duty. The spots were not indeed at that time quite off his body, nor his gums sound; but without any other medicine, than a gargarism of elixir vitriol, he became quite healthy before we came into Plymouth, which was on 16 June. The other was the best recovered of any in his condition; and being now deemed pretty well, was appointed nurse to the rest of the sick.

Next to the oranges, I thought the cider had the best effects. It was indeed not very sound, being inclinable to be eager or pricked. However, those who had taken it, were in a fairer way of recovery than the others at the end of the fortnight, which was the length of time all these different courses were continued, except the oranges. The putrefaction of their gums, but especially their lassitude and weakness, were somewhat abated, and their appetite increased by it.

As to the elixir of vitriol, I observed that the mouths of those who had used it by way of gargarism, were in a much cleaner and better condition than many of the rest, especially those who used the vinegar; but perceived otherwise no good effects from its internal use upon the other symptoms. [. . .]

There was no remarkable alteration upon those who took the electuary and tamarind decoction, the sea-water, or vinegar, upon comparing their condition, at the end of the fortnight, with others who had taken nothing but a little lenitive electuary and *cremor tartar*, [. . .].

I cannot omit upon this occasion observing, what caution is at all times necessary in our reasoning on the effects of medicines, even in the way of analogy, which would seem the least liable to error. For some might naturally conclude that these fruits are but so many acids, for which tamarinds, vinegar, *sp. sal.*, *el. vitriol*, and others of the same tribe, would prove excellent *succedaneums*. But upon bringing this to the test of experience, we find the contrary. Few ships have ever been in want of vinegar, and, for many years before the end of the late war, all were supplied sufficiently with *el. vitriol*. Notwithstanding which, the Channel fleet often put on shore a thousand men miserably over-run with this disease, besides some hundreds who died in their cruises. Upon those occasions tar-water, salt water, vinegar, and *el. vitriol* especially, with many other things, have been abundantly tried to no purpose: whereas there is not an instance of a ship's crew being over afflicted with this disease, where the before mentioned fruits were properly, duly, and in sufficient quantity, administered.

[. . .]

Some will perhaps say, that these fruits have been often used in the scurvy without success; as appears from the experience of physicians, who prescribe them every day in that disease at land. And here we may again observe the fatal consequences of confounding this malady with others. Legions of distempers (according to Willis and others) very different from the real and genuine scurvy, have been classed under its name: and because the most approved antiscorbutics fail to remove such diseases, hence we are told by authors that it is the masterpiece of art to cure it. But this is contradicted by the daily experience of seamen, by the journals of our sea-hospitals, and by the yearly experience of our English East-India ships at St Helena, and the Cape of Good Hope. So that nothing can be more absurd, than to object against the efficacy of these fruits in preventing and curing the real scurvy, because they do not cure very different diseases.

John Hunter

John Hunter, one of the important builders of modern medicine, was born in Scotland in 1728. His brother William, older by ten years, had achieved substantial success in London as an anatomist and obstetrician, and had established a dissecting academy. John went to London, worked with his brother and acquired great skill in anatomy. While engaged in anatomical teaching and investigation, John also studied in London hospitals. In 1760 he joined the army and saw service in foreign campaigns. Returning to London in 1763, he engaged in surgical practice and in anatomical and physiological researches. His surgical skill brought him both fame and a substantial income, most of which he spent on his superb natural history museum where he carried out much of his investigative work. He died in 1793.

Hunter was an extraordinarily versatile person, whose interests ranged widely over the whole field of biology and medicine. Possessed of insatiable curiosity, he was constantly asking questions and, even more important, constantly trying to find the answers. Asking questions is easy, but seeking the answers by one's own effort is relatively rare. John Hunter had this trait to a marked degree.

Not content to make observations in a merely passive fashion he engaged actively in experimentation to help him answer specific questions. But his interests ranged so widely that his investigations were rather diffuse. He covered a great variety of topics but did not pursue any of them with the single-minded intensity that we see in some researchers. Unfortunately, his gifts as a naturalist and experimental biologist did not extend to the field of self-expression. While Hunter's writings are sometimes relatively clear, for the most part his thought is badly expressed.

He did not try to make complex hypotheses nor form systems nor provide overall explanations. He remained quite close to concrete observations, tried to expand them by experiment and to show how new facts entered into relationship with other facts. From these interrelationships he drew cautious conclusions. He did not have a speculative bent, nor any interest in metaphysics or over-arching theory.

His writings are full of interesting observations and discussions, with narrative accounts of particular problems and the steps he took to find solutions. A good example, taken from the *Treatise on the Blood, Inflammation, and Gunshot Wounds*, has to do with the colour of the blood. Venous blood is dark, and arterial blood is florid. What factors produce the change from one to the other? Hunter devised suitable experiments to throw light on these questions.

When reading the excerpts bearing on the problem, we must remember that he held some beliefs about blood that sound odd to us today. Hunter thought that the blood was 'alive'. He did not try to define that term with any precision, and his numerous references to the life in blood do not affect his methodology.

From his various experimental studies he concluded that during life the dark colour of the blood correlated with a slowing down of the motion of the blood. The question as to whether the blood was arterial or venous was not so important, for under suitable circumstances arterial blood could be dark, venous blood florid. The speed of motion was important.

John Hunter represented the empirical trend in eighteenth-century medicine, in contrast to a systematist and rationalist trend that engaged so many physicians. In the present volume of selections we can place Hunter in the same category as Morgagni and Lind, and contrast these three with Hoffmann, Boerhaave and Cullen, leading systematists of the era.

12 A Treatise on the Blood, Inflammation and Gunshot Wounds (1794)

Excerpts from J. Hunter, *A Treatise on The Blood, Inflammation, and Gunshot Wounds*, James Webster, 1817, pp. 47–53.

I put some dark venal blood into a phial, till it was about half full, and shook the blood, which mixed with the air in this motion, and it became immediately of a florid red.

[. . .]

The blood of the menses, when it comes down to the mouth of the vagina, is as dark as venal blood; and as it does not coagulate, it has exactly the appearance of the blood in those where the blood continues fluid. Whether this arises from its being venal blood, or from its acquiring that colour after extravasation, by its slow motion, it is not easily determined; but upon being exposed it becomes florid: it is naturally of a dark colour, but rather muddy, not having that transparency which pure blood has. Whether this arises from its mixing with the mucus of the vagina, or from the cessation of life in it, I will not pretend to say. [. . .]

The surface of the blood becoming of a scarlet red, whether exposed immediately to the air, or when only covered by membranes, through which we may suppose its influence to pass, is a circumstance which leads us to suppose, that it is the pure air which has this effect, and not simply an exposed surface. To ascertain this, I made the following experiment.

I took a phial, and fixed a stop-cock to its mouth, and then applying an air-pump to the cock, exhausted the whole air; in this state keeping it stopped, I immersed its mouth in fresh blood flowing from a vein, and then turning the cock, allowed the blood to be pressed up into the phial. When it was about half full, I turned the cock back, and now shook the phial with the blood, but its colour did not alter, as in the former experiments; and when I allowed the blood to stand in this vacuum, its exposed surface was not in the least changed.

[. . .]

I have shown that several substances mixed with dark coloured blood, have the property of rendering it of a florid red; and it must have appeared, that by circulating through the body, its dark colour is restored. As it is capable of being rendered florid, by several substances, so it may be rendered dark by several when florid: vital air has the power of rendering it florid; but the other vapours, or gases, which have the name of airs, such as fixed air, inflammable air, etc. render it dark. This change is peculiar to the living body; for if arterial blood is taken away, it retains its florid colour, although not in the least exposed to the air. As it is found dark in the veins, and as it performs some offices in the course of the circulation, which perhaps render it unfit for the purposes of life, we may conceive that the loss of colour, and this unfitness, are effects of the same cause: but, upon further observations on this fluid, it will be found that it may be rendered unfit for the purposes of life, without losing its colour; and may lose its colour without being rendered unfit for life: slowness of motion in the blood of the veins, is one circumstance that causes the alteration; but this alone will not produce the effect; for I have observed above that arterial blood put into a phial, and allowed to stand quiet, does not become dark; but rest, or slowness of motion in living parts, would appear, from many observations, to be a cause of this change in its colour: we know that the blood begins to move more and more slowly in the arteries: we know its motion in the veins is slow, in comparison to what it is in the arteries; we should, therefore, naturally suppose, (considering this alone) that it was the slowness of the motion that was the immediate cause. Rest, or slowness of motion, in living, and probably healthy parts, certainly allows the blood to change its colour: thus we never see extravasations of blood, but it is continually dark. I never saw a person die of an apoplexy, from extravasation in the brain, but the extravasated blood was dark; even in aneurysm it becomes dark in the aneurysmal sac; also when the blood escapes out of the artery, and coagulates in the cellular membrane, we find the same appearance.

These observations respecting apoplexy struck me much. I conceived at first that the extravasations there must consist of venal blood; but, from reasoning, I could hardly allow myself to think so; for whatever might be the beginning of the disease, it was impossible it could continue afterwards wholly venal; especially when the blood was found in a considerable quantity; because, in many cases, great mischief was done to both systems of vessels, and the arteries once ruptured would give the greatest quantity of blood; but to ascertain this with more certainty, I made the following experiment:

I wounded the femoral artery of a puppy obliquely; the opening in the skin was made at some distance from the artery, by a couching needle; the blood that came from the small orifice in the skin was florid. The cellular membrane swelled up very much; about five minutes afterwards, I punctured the tumour, and the blood was fluid. In ten minutes I punctured it again; the blood was thinner, and more serous, but still florid. In fifteen minutes I punctured it again: at first only serum issued; upon squeezing, a little blood came, but still florid: the mass now seemed to be principally coagulated, which prevented further trials. Some days after, when I cut into the swelled part, I found the blood as dark as common venal blood; so that here the change had taken place after coagulation.

When I had plaster of Paris applied to my face to make a mould, in the taking it off, it produced a kind of suction on the fore part of the nose, which I felt; and when the plaster was removed, on observing the part, it was red, as if the cells of the skin were loaded with extravasated blood; this was then of a florid red, but it soon became of a dark purple, which showed that it was arterial blood, and that by stagnating in the cells of the body it became of the colour of venal blood.

Blood may even be rendered dark in the larger arteries, by a short stagnation. I laid bare the carotid artery of a dog, for about two inches in length; I then tied a thread round it at each end, leaving a space of two inches in length between each ligature, filled with blood; the external wound was stitched loosely up: several hours after, I opened the stitches, and observed in this vessel that the blood was coagulated, and of a dark colour, the same as in the vein. Thus I have also seen when a tourniquet has been applied round the thigh, and the artery divided, that when it was slackened the first blood came out of a dark colour, but what followed was florid.

This I have seen in amputations, when a tourniquet had been

applied for a considerable time; and it is commonly observed in performing the operation for the aneurism.

July, 1779, Mr Bromfield had a patient in St George's Hospital, with an aneurism in the crural artery, about the middle of the thigh; the artery had been dilated about three inches in length. The operation was performed, in which the artery was tied up above the dilatation, three or more inches, for security. When this was done, the tourniquet was slackened, and a pretty considerable bleeding was observed, seemingly at the lower orifice, leading from the dilated part, which, at first, was supposed from its colour, to be the venous blood that had stagnated in the veins, by means of the tourniquet; but this it could not be; and it was found to flow from the lower orifice of the artery, which was immediately tied: we must suppose, that the motion of the blood, in making this retrogade course, was very slow; for it had first to pass off into small collateral branches, above where it was tied, then to anastomose with similar small ones, from the trunk below, and then to enter that trunk; all of which must very much retard its motion; and, indeed, the manner of its oozing out of the vessels showed such a retardation. This motion of the blood, though in the arterial system, was in some respects similar to the motion of the blood in both systems of vessels.

This last circumstance plainly indicates a communication of the arteries above the aneurism with those below, by means of the anastomosing branches.

The blood from the lower orifice flowed without any pulsation; which must have been owing to its coming into the large artery below by a vast number of smaller ones at different distances, and of course at different times; but probably, the chief cause of this want of pulsation in the great artery was, that the power of the heart was lost in the two systems of smaller arteries above and below; for the second system, or those from below, became in a considerable degree similar to veins; and the great artery in the leg below the aneurism was like a considerable vein.

A young man, servant to Henry Drummond, Esq., having had a knife run into his thigh, which wounded the crural artery, a considerable tumour came on the part, consisting chiefly of blood extravasated, and lodged in the cellular membrane. This in some degree stopped the flowing of the blood from the cut artery, and on dilating the wound so as to get to the artery, I observed that the extravasated blood in the cellular membrane was of the venal colour. On exposing the artery, which was first secured from bleeding by a tourniquet above, and then slightly slackening that instrument, the first blood which flowed from above was dark, and even was taken for venous blood by the operator; but he was soon cónvinced that it was arterial, by the florid colour of that which almost immediately ensued. I observed that the colour of the blood was as dark as that of any venous blood I ever saw.

From these experiments, and observation, we must conclude that the colour of the blood is altered, either by rest, or slow motion, in living parts, and even in the arteries; this circumstance takes place in the vessels as the motion of the blood decreases.

Another observation occurs, viz. that the whole of the limbs below the ligature, where the crural artery has been taken up, must be entirely supplied with such altered blood; and as this leg kept its life, its warmth, and the action of the muscles, it is evident that the colour of the blood is of little service to any of those properties.

[. . .]

Another observation strongly in favour of the supposition that rest is a cause of the change of blood from the scarlet colour to the dark, or modena, is taken from the common operation of bleeding; for we generally find the blood of a dark colour at its first coming out, but it becomes lighter and lighter towards the last. Some reason may be given for this: first, it has stagnated in the veins, while the vein was filling, and the orifice making, which occupies some time, and may render it darker than it otherwise might have been in the same vein: secondly, when there is a free orifice, the blood may pass more readily into the veins from the arteries, and therefore may be somewhat in the state of arterial blood, which may occasion the last blood to be rather lighter.

Giovanni Battista Morgagni

Morgagni lived a long and remarkably full life. As a youth he was precocious and as an old man he preserved his acumen and energy and, indeed, published his greatest work when he was seventy-nine. He was born in 1682 in Forli, received his medical degree in 1701 from Bologna, and became professor of practical medicine at Padua in 1711. Four years later, appointed professor of anatomy of that university, he occupied the chair held by such medical pathfinders as Vesalius, Realdus Columbus and Fallopius.

Morgagni was a clinician, anatomist and pathologist, but his great reputation rests upon his pathology text, *The Seats and Causes of Diseases Investigated by Anatomy*, published in Latin in 1761. At this time there were no professional pathologists in the modern sense, no men who devoted themselves entirely to the study of 'morbid anatomy'. Pathology was a part-time activity and the dissections to discover the cause of death were performed by clinicians and anatomists. Such dissections were frequently undertaken.

In 1679 a large number of autopsy reports were compiled by Bonetus. This collection, the *Sepulchretum*, constituted a great landmark in pathology. It brought together the autopsy findings in a wide range of conditions. While this book reveals the great variety of conditions studied, it had relatively little to say about each case. The examinations were carried out with varying degrees of thoroughness, and even the longest and most detailed descriptions were relatively cursory. Distinctions between pathological findings and post-mortem artifacts were not made. And the post-mortem examinations, for the most part, did not have any clinical information, at least not enough to make significant correlation with the anatomical findings.

Morgagni, on the other hand, was a superb observer, careful and precise, who went into great and sometimes wearisome detail. He recognized that real progress could come only by correlating anatomical findings and clinical manifestations. The mere fact that a cadaver showed this or that discolouration or swelling or softening or collection of fluid had little significance unless it were tied together with appearances during life, and the clinical course of the disease.

In his book he collected a great many cases – some from his own practice, some from his teacher Fallopius, and some from other clinicians as well – and emphasized the symptomatology, clinical course and therapy, and then the post-mortem findings. Then he tried to correlate the two series of events and show how the morphologic alterations of disease accounted for the symptoms. We must remember, of course, that compared with modern pathologists he was quite ignorant of disease states, and the complex interrelations of morphology and function. With no microscopic examinations to help him, he was dependent entirely on gross observation. Within the limits of knowledge then available, he did an excellent and illuminating correlative study.

The quotations given illustrate three separate diseases. One is a case of lobar pneumonia. It would be well for the reader to compare his description of the clinical appearances with Cullen's description of the stages of fever. In the second case, a ruptured aneurysm of the aorta, the interest rests on the clinical aspect and on therapy. He had already described numerous cases of aneurysm, in many of which he discussed the pathogenesis at length. The third case was a pericardial effusion, where the correlations between the clinical aspects and the pathologic findings are by no means entirely satisfactory. We feel that the pathologic descriptions are quite inadequate. But the case has particular interest for showing the clinical approach to an obscure case, the attempt to analyse the pathophysiology while the patient was still alive, and the interest in performing the autopsy examination to elucidate the problem.

It would be quite misleading to choose only cases where the diagnosis accorded with modern views and the descriptions were consonant with modern concepts. The three cases exhibit not only a range of conditions, but a range of knowledge and a variety of approach. They provide a good view of the best eighteenth-century practice.

13 The Seats and Causes of Disease (1769)

Excerpts from J. B. Morgagni, *The Seats and Causes of Diseases Investigated by Anatomy*, vol. 1, translated by Benjamin Alexander, Nullar, 1769, pp. 604–6, 796–7, 412–14.

Book II Of Diseases of the Thorax

Letter XXI

26. Now I will pass over from this kind of epidemic inflammation of the lungs, which raged at that time among the poor at Bologna, to another at Padua, which spread about in the winter of the year 1738; and nowhere more than in some convents of nuns, and especially in one, to such a degree, that all who were seized with it died, and some even within four days. Which was the reason, without doubt, that, as nine had already died, I was publicly commanded to enquire into the nature of the disease, even by dissection. It was not difficult to conceive, that there was nothing contagious in it, as none of those who had attended upon the sick had contracted the disease, and even they, who had taken the most care to keep themselves from them, were seized with it; but not without a peculiar cause, and disposition, in almost every one. One of them, for instance, had had an ulcer of long standing in her leg, which was now healed up; another had had a previous fall upon her chest, and had spit a great quantity of blood in this last sickness; another had been long inclined to a pulmonary phthisis; and in fine, others had other causes to render the powers of the thorax and lungs infirm, as they who were of a decrepit age.

But nevertheless, although out of those who had been ill at that time, notwithstanding three different physicians had been employed, some having been attended by one, and some by another, not one could be saved, as I have said; yet by many this was not ascribed so much to the violence of the disorder, as to its nature not being well known, and especially by the inhabitants of the convent. And by what means I exorted this judgment from them, you will know from the subjoined history. For when the tenth was now dead, and those physicians and I came together to the dissection of her, I begged of them, before the dissection was begun, that they would relate what had been observed, and what had been done, in the disorder. Which the senior physician who had attended upon her, did very accurately in the manner I shall relate presently; the others at the same time affirming, that they also had seen, and done, almost the same things, in the others, except that one, who had given fresh-drawn oil of almonds, ingenuously added, that the patient had been worse from it. But let us come to her who was then to be dissected.

27. A virgin, of two-and-forty years of age, who had, every winter, been subject to a violent cough, of a very good habit of body, and abounding in blood, being employed in great and continual labours for the service of the convent, was seized in the night with a fever, with which she first shivered, and was cold through her whole body, and after that grew hot. After an interval of twenty-four hours, a pain on one side of the breast was added to the fever, together with a difficulty of breathing, a cough quite dry, and a rather hard pulse, which resisted the pressure of the fingers, even almost to the very time of the patient's death. In the progress of the disease, the pain shifted from one side of the breast to the opposite part. There was a sense of weight within the thorax. She could lie down upon neither side. In the blood that was taken from her the serum was of a greenish colour, there was a polypus crust, and the other part of it, that lay under this, had a very great blackness and hardness. And blood was taken away immediately as the pain came on, and after that once, and even twice, in a proper quantity, for a body of that kind; and not only from the arms, but from the feet also, within the same day, as the custom always is here, in regard to women. Nor was any thing omitted besides, of all the remedies customary in disorders of this kind. Nevertheless, on the beginning of the seventh day she died. When I had heard this relation, I said, in dependance upon those appearances, that I had always found after the chief of such kind of symptoms, 'Come, let the body be dissected; this will be certainly found to be the nature of the disease, that the lungs shall appear to have the substance of the liver.'

In the thorax, then, when opened by the surgeon, there was no extravasated humour, and no connection of the lungs with the pleura, except at the left side; and this was neither very close, nor to any considerable extent. While this connection was disjoined, and the lungs, on that account, pressed, a turbid serum flowed out, in some considerable quantity; but whether from the lungs, as it seemed to us, or from the interstice left between this and the pleura, within the borders of the connection, was the more uncertain, as neither the lungs, nor the pleura, in that place, showed any particular injury; but the lungs were covered with a whitish and thickish kind of membrane, such as I have often described in the foregoing histories, even where the lungs were quite free; and to the corresponding pleura, quite upon the surface, adhered a reddish kind of sediment, such as would subside in water wherein fresh meat had been washed. In another place, where there had been no adhesion, the surface of the lungs was prominent into a kind of tubercle, which being cut into, discharged a whitish kind of serum like pus. We then ordered the lungs to be taken out, and they were not only heavy, but, in more than one place, hard. When they were cut into, they appeared to have a dense and compact substance, like that of the liver, as I had predicted, and not only on the surface, but to great depths internally, being in other parts, in general, of a redder complexion, and abounding with that whitish serum which was found in the tubercle; and from hence it was very evident, that the inflammation of both lobes of the lungs, which already degenerated into suppuration, had been the cause of her death. However, in the pericardium was scarcely any serum; and in the heart no polypus concretion was found; because the left ventricle contained scarcely any blood, and the right only a little more, which was black, and not at all fluid.

28. Having found these appearances, I returned, together with the other physicians, to the place where we were expected by the abbess, and said to her, It is not an unknown and a rare disorder, as you was afraid, which has carried off so many virgins; but the vehemence of one that is very common, and very well known. And to convince you that it is really so, I foretold, previously to the dissection of the body, that the lungs would be found to be in such a state, as they were really found to be in; and this it would have been impossible for me to have done, if I had not very

frequently dissected those, who died of this disorder: and I did it on purpose, that you yourselves might readily understand that to be true, which I just now pronounced. By this means they were freed from their fears, and their opinions of the disease being unknown; and our discourse was turned to propose that method, which has turned out most successfully, by which the other nuns, and especially those who had their lungs very lax, and weak, might beware of the disease; for it did not seem at all doubtful to us, but that the peripneumony could not be overcome in those who had died, chiefly for this cause.

[. . .]

Letter XXVI

9. A man who had been too much given to the exercise of tennis and the abuse of wine, was, in consequence of both these irregularities, seized with a pain of the right arm, and soon after of the left, joined with a fever. After these there appeared a tumour on the upper part of the sternum, like a large boil: by which appearance some vulgar surgeons being deceived, and either not having at all observed, or having neglected, the pulsation, applied such things as are generally used to bring these tumours to suppuration; and these applications were of the most violent kind. As the tumour still increased, others applied emollient medicines, from which it seemed to them to be diminished; that is, from the fibres being rubbed with ointments and relaxed; whereas they had been before greatly irritated by the applications. But as this circumstance related rather to the common integuments, than to the tumour itself, or to the coats that were proper thereto, it not only soon recovered its former magnitude, but even was plainly seen to increase every day. Wherefore, when the patient came into the Hospital of Incurables, at Bologna, which was, I suppose, in the year 1704, it was equal in size to a quince; and what was much worse, it began to exude blood in one place; so that the man himself was very near having broken through the skin (this being reduced to the utmost thinness in that part, and he being quite ignorant of the danger which was at hand) when he began to pull off the bandages, for the sake of showing his disorder. But this circumstance being observed, he was prevented going on, and ordered to keep him-

self still, and to think seriously and piously of his departure from this mortal life, which was very near at hand, and inevitable. And this really happened on the day following, from the vast profusion of blood that had been foretold, though not so soon expected by the patient. Nevertheless, he had the presence of mind, immediately as he felt the blood gushing forth, not only to commend himself to God, but to take up with his own hands a basin that lay at his bedside; and, as if he had been receiving the blood of another person, put it beneath the gaping tumour, while the attendants immediately ran to him as fast as possible, in whose arms he soon after expired.

In examining the body before I dissected it, I saw that there was no longer any tumour, inasmuch as it had subsided after the blood, by which it had been raised up externally, had been discharged. The skin was there broken through, and the parts that lie beneath it with an aperture, which admitted two fingers at once. The *membrana adiposa* of the thorax discharged a water during the time of dissection, with which some vessels were also turgid, that were prominent, here and there, upon the surface of the skin in the feet and the legs. In both the cavities of the thorax, also, was a great quantity of water, of a yellowish colour. And there was a large aneurysm, into which the anterior part of the curvature of the aorta itself being expanded, had partly consumed the upper part of the sternum, the extremities of the clavicles which lie upon it and the neighbouring ribs, and partly had made them diseased, by bringing on a caries. And where the bones had been consumed or affected with the caries, there not the least traces of the coats of the artery remained: to which, in other places, a thick substance every where adhered internally, resembling a dry and lurid kind of flesh, distinguished with some whitish points; and this substance you might easily divide into many membranes, as it were, one lying upon another, quite different in their nature from those coats to which they adhered, as they were evidently polypus. And these things being accurately attended to, nothing occurred besides that was worthy of remark.

10. The deplorable exit of this man teaches, in the first place, how much care ought to be taken in the beginning, that an internal aneurysm may obtain no increase: and in the second place, if,

either by the ignorance of the persons who attempt their cure, or the disobedience of the patient, or only by the force of the disorder itself, they do at length increase, so that they are only covered by the common integuments of the whole body; that then we ought to take care lest the bandages, especially when they are already dried to the part, be hastily taken off: and finally, if the case proceed to such an extremity, that the rupture of the skin is every day impending, and bleeding, either on account of the constitution or infirmity of the patient, or on the score of other things which I have hinted at already, is dangerous; that everything is to be previously studied, by which, for some days at least, life may be prolonged. That is to say, besides the greatest tranquillity of body and of mind, and the greatest abstinence that can be consistently observed, so that no more food be taken than is barely necessary for the preservation of life, and that in small quantities, and of such a quality as is by no means stimulating; besides that situation of body; by which the weight of the blood being lessened, does not press upon the skin, and other things of the like kind; something ought to be thought of by the surgeon, by way of defence; as, for instance, if the bladder of an ox, four times doubled, were applied, or a bandage of soft leather; and the edges of this bandage were all daubed over with a medicine, by which they would be firmly glued down to the neighbouring skin that lay around the tumour, and was as yet sound and entire. But you will judge better of these things; for as to me, carried away with a desire of preserving a man's life, though but for one short hour, I perhaps talk foolishly. As to straight bandages, and plates of elastic steel or the like, I say nothing of them; not so much on account of those things which Lancisi has observed, of the most considerable injuries being brought on by them in process of time; for the question is not at present how the patient may live the longest time he possible can, but only how to prevent his dying immediately; as on account of the skin being extenuated, in which case all pressure is dangerous. [. . .]

Letter XVI

43. There was at Bologna a nun, whose illustrious family and convent I might mention here, if I chose it, whom a physician had cured of a defluxion upon her gums and cheeks, by giving

her sudorific decoctions of the woods; and afterwards, being seized with an acute fever, had restored to health with equal success. Though he might have been content with one and the other of these successful cures, yet, as some are diligent to a very ill purpose, when the month of April returned, he began to urge this virgin, that she should not let slip a time so opportune for the taking of those remedies by which she had preserved herself from the defluxions. She at first refused to comply, inasmuch as she was in very good health, and thought her constitution sufficiently altered and rectified by the decoction and the fever together; yet as the man very often inculcated the necessity of such a treatment, she at length consented, but unwillingly, as if her mind had, in some measure, presaged what would happen; for having taken as much of the same *syrupus aureus*, as it is called, as others in the convent had taken on that very day, with every one of whom it had succeeded extremely well; with her, whatever was the cause of so unexpected an accident, it occasioned near fifty motions of stool; by which as generally happens after a great quantity of serum being discharged, an intolerable thirst was brought on, that did not remit upon drinking a very large quantity of broths; and, for this reason, the physician ordered her to drink a very large quantity of dilute emulsions; nor did the quantity of urine that she made, answer at all to the quantity of fluid she took in. The day afterwards, having sat up in bed, with an intention to rise, and having begun to put on her clothes, she was suddenly seized with a kind of oppression at her heart, to which a fainting fit succeeded; and from that time, this oppression never failed to be exacerbated as often as ever she spoke or moved too much. Many physicians were sent for, whose opinions, as generally happens in disorders of this kind, being very different from one another, Albertini was added to their number. It was now the month of July: when they came together, one began to conjecture a polypus, another an aneurysm, another a tubercle of the lungs; nor were they wanting who had a suspicion of a dropsy of the lungs, or the thorax. When it came to Albertini to give his opinion (whose cautious delay in this case I was always better pleased to imitate, rather than the bold hastiness of some) he affirmed that it did not become his modesty to undertake to determine immediately, from having seen the patient but once, what so many men, excelling in years, authority, learning, ingenuity and experience, could not sufficiently have determined upon in almost three months; and begged, therefore, that they would permit him, by visiting the patient once or twice more, to endeavour to find out the nature of so obscure a disorder, which he should perhaps better understand from what he might see than from what he had heard, and after visiting the patient diligently several times, and considering not only the symptoms that were present, but what were absent also, with great attention, he called together again the council of physicians, and first gave them his reasons one by one, why it seemed less probable to him that the disorder was of the kind any of them had mentioned, than that it was a dropsy, and that of the pericardium: a dropsy surely, for it had taken its origin immediately from the time of so much water being carried into the constitution, which had neither been discharged again from the body, nor could in so short a time have been mixed with the blood; for which reason, a portion of it must be supposed to have fallen upon some part or other, that by the original constitution, as frequently happens, was more disposed to suffer it than other parts; and that the dropsy was of the pericardium, because he had found by dissection, that some had had water collected in that cavity, in whom he had observed the same, or similar symptoms while living.

Attend now to those disagreeable symptoms that did not exist in this virgin. She had a good colour in her face; her sleep was undisturbed; she was regular in her bowels, and in her menstrua; her respiration was equally easy, whether she stood up or lay on her back, on the right or on the left side. Her pulse was neither tense, nor hard, nor chord-like, nor in the least irregular in any way. She had no palpitation, or large pulsation, in the heart; no pain about the region of the lungs; no cough; there was not the least thing, if you except what I have said above, and what I shall say presently, there was nothing, I say, that you could find fault with, or that she could complain of. Albertini, being persuaded by these arguments, did not fall into the opinion of others. And he thought that these signs had a tendency to confirm his opinion, that the virgin found her heart oppressed, as if with a stone being laid upon it; and that when she did not speak, and was quiet, and free from motion, she was not troubled with that oppression of the heart, as I mentioned in the beginning; but if she performed any motion, or spoke for any little time, she was immediately tortured therewith, the sensation of which she used to express thus, as if she was pressed and squeezed up, with a great concourse of people all round her: and this oppression of her heart, a slight kind of fainting always accompanied; and her pulse, even when she was quiet, was always weak. Which circumstances certainly rendered the cure very difficult; for besides that if by medicines they should attempt to discharge the collected serum, there was danger, lest that being rather diminished, which is necessary to the blood, the circulation should be carried on with much more difficulty through the heart, which was compressed by the water, and already flaccid by its long stagnation; this was certainly very evident, that whatever remedies were very efficacious, would without doubt have the same effect upon her as the motion of her body had; and those that were less efficacious, would be of no use at all, or at least not sufficiently advantageous. This was actually the case; and the virgin at length died of the disorder, as Albertini had predicted when he considered these things. For when she had dragged on life, to about the end of a year from the beginning of her disease, a momentary sense of pricking began to be added to the other symptoms, which returned every now and then in the part affected, attended with slight convulsions in the same place; the pulse began gradually to be more and more weakened, and in a manner obscured; which were not fallacious symptoms of death being now at hand.

It was permitted to Albertini to open the thorax in order to discover the nature of so abstruse a disease, Robert Muratorio, a senior physician, and an eminent man, being added as his only companion in the dissection. Everything was found to be found, and in proper condition, except that the pericardium was tumid with water, to the quantity of nine ounces, and the membrane of the heart had begun to be evidently eroded, without doubt from the same water, which was at length become very acrid from its stagnation, from whence that sense of pricking had been felt, and those slight convulsions had happened.

Marie-François-Xavier Bichat

One of the great figures in medical history, Marie-François-Xavier Bichat died at the early age of thirty-one. His entire medical career, from the time he first began his medical studies until his death in 1802, spanned only eleven years, yet in this short interval he helped to mould medical theory.

His life mirrored the turbulence of the French Revolution. Born in 1771, he started to study medicine at Lyons, but the revolutionary disturbances forced him to flee to Paris in 1793. Here he was befriended by the surgeon Desault, whose favourite pupil he became. When Desault died prematurely in 1795, Bichat collected and edited his master's works, In addition, he lectured and taught, carried out his own researches, worked prodigiously in the clinical wards, the dissecting rooms, and the laboratory, and also wrote extensively. He died quite suddenly of what is thought to be tuberculous meningitis. His major works were the *Traité sur les membranes* and the *Recherches physiologiques sur la vie et sur la mort*, published in 1800, and the *Anatomie générale* the next year. His *Anatomie descriptive*, published in part in 1801, was completed posthumously by friends.

Bichat did not make any great discoveries, but he helped to create and popularize important attitudes which affected the whole current of medical thought. We can indicate several features that in a sense complement each other. First of all, he stressed the characteristic 'vital' properties in living creatures, properties which he maintained were completely different from those of brute and inert matter. Regarding living organisms as quite distinct from the non-living, he contrasted organic with inorganic, vital with non-vital, physiological with physical. Just as the physical world had its 'first principles' such as gravity, so the physiological world had its basic or ultimate principles of sensibility and contractility. He was thus an extreme vitalist who continued the tradition of Stahl that had already been strengthened by the physicians of Montpellier. While his views no longer have any cogency, they did set biology apart from any crude mechanistic interpretation.

His emphasis on the analytic viewpoint was a second major contribution. Whereas previous pathologists and clinicians had considered the organs as the basis of normal function and of disease process, Bichat carried the analysis much further. Organs had their components – the tissues – and by distinguishing these components from each other, he could make much finer discriminations and much more precise correlations between pathologic changes and clinical symptomatology. Interestingly enough, although he has been called the Father of Histology, he did not use the microscope, but for his analytic tools depended on simple experimental procedures employing physical and chemical agents.

In addition, Bichat greatly advanced the empirical and experimental viewpoints. A tireless worker, he stressed observation and experiment but at the same time worked within the framework of his vitalistic concepts. Theory dominated his overall approach and led to concrete observations, to questions asked of nature, and to techniques for finding the answers. If we compare him with John Hunter we find many similarities, but Bichat had the greater theoretical insight and the more comprehensive approach that theory provides.

A further contribution we find in his positivistic attitude towards experiment. His vitalistic biology was in no way obscurantist or mystical. He was not concerned with metaphysical essence or 'inner' nature of things, but rather with observable phenomena and what could be inferred from them. He held that we must study observable reactions; through these reactions we make discriminations without worrying about hidden essences. In this regard he reminds us of Sydenham.

The quotations given here, in my own translation, are taken from the preface of the *Anatomie générale*. The excerpts reveal some of his basic principles, both of theory and of methodology.

14 General Anatomy (1801)

Excerpts from M.-F.-X. Bichat, *Anatomie Générale, Appliquée à la Physiologie et à la Médecine*, vol. 1, Brosson, Gabon et Cie, 1801, translated by Lester S. King, preface, pp. li–xciv.

In nature there are two classes of being, two classes of properties, two classes of science. Beings are either organic or inorganic; the properties, vital or non-vital (living or non-living); the sciences, physiological or physical. Animals and vegetables are organic, while what we call the mineral kingdom is inorganic. Sensibility and contractility are the vital properties. Gravity, affinity, elasticity, and the like, represent the non-vital properties. Animal physiology, plant physiology, and medicine comprise the physiological sciences. Astronomy, physics, chemistry, and the like, are the physical sciences [. . .].

Characteristics of vital properties, compared with physical properties

[. . .] Physical laws are constant and invariable, not subject either to increase or decrease. In no case does a stone gravitate toward the centre of the earth with greater force than ordinary; in no case does marble have greater elasticity, and so on. On the other hand, [in the organic world] at each moment the sensibility and the contractility may change and become greater or less. They are almost never the same.

It follows that physical phenomena are entirely invariable; that at all periods, and under all influences, they are the same. Consequently we can foresee, predict and calculate them [. . .]. Once the formula has been found, we need only apply it to every case [. . .]. All vital functions, on the contrary, undergo a host of variations. Frequently they depart from their natural states; they elude any kind of calculation; there would necessarily be almost as many formulae as cases in hand. We can foresee nothing, predict nothing for their phenomena. We have only approximation, and most often uncertain at that.

Vital phenomena show two aspects – a state of health and a state of disease – and hence two distinct sciences – physiology, concerned with phenomena of the first category, and pathology, with the second. The [natural] history of phenomena wherein vital forces exhibit their natural character leads to the study of phenomena where these forces are altered. But in the physical sciences we have only the first type of history; the second is never encountered. Physiology has the same relation to the movements of living body as astronomy, dynamics, hydraulics, hydrostatics, etc., have to movements of inert bodies. For these latter there are no sciences corresponding to pathology of living bodies. By the same token, any concept of therapeutics is entirely foreign to the physical sciences. A therapeutic substance has as its goal the restoration of properties to their natural type. But physical properties never depart from their type, and do not have any need to be restored thereto. In the physical sciences nothing corresponds to the place of therapeutics in physiology. We see, then, how the special character of instability in the vital properties produces an enormous series of phenomena requiring a quite special kind of science. What would become of the world if the laws of physics were subjected to the same disturbances, to the same variations as vital laws? [. . .]

Just as the phenomena and the laws are so different in the physical and the physiological sciences, so these sciences themselves must have essential differences. The way of presenting the facts and of searching out their causes, and the modes of experiment, must have a quite different character. It is a mistake to confuse these sciences. Inasmuch as the physical sciences were perfected before the physiological ones, men thought to clarify the latter by associating them with the former, but have succeeded only in confusing them. This was inevitable, for to apply physical sciences to physiology is to explain the phenomena of living bodies by the laws of inert bodies. This is a false principle, and everything derived therefrom is similarly incorrect. Leave to the chemist his affinity, to the physicist his elasticity and gravity. For physiology use only sensibility and contractility. I make exception of the cases where a single organ is the seat of both vital and physical phenomena, such as the eye and the ear, for example. [. . .]

The works of Stahl have the real advantage of disregarding all these supposed accessory aids, which crush the science while wishing to support it. But, as this great physician had not analysed the vital properties, he could not present the phenomena under their true aspect. Nothing is more vague and uncertain than such words as 'vitality', 'vital influx', and the like, when their meaning has not been rigorously defined. Suppose that in the physical sciences someone had thought up some general and vague words which alone correspond to all the non-vital properties, which provide only ideas that are general and not at all precise. If you introduce such words, if you do not clarify what belongs to gravity, what depends on affinity, what is the result of elasticity, and so on, you will never be understood. Let us say as much for the physiological sciences. [. . .]

Look at the solid parts of the living body, incessantly building up and breaking down, every moment taking and rejecting new substances. The inert solids, on the contrary, remain inert, constantly the same, preserving the same elements until friction or other causes destroy them. Similarly, you see in the elements of inert fluids an unchanging uniformity, a constant identity in their principles which are known as soon as they have been analysed a single time. The principles which vary incessantly in the fluids of the living body require a host of analyses, performed under all possible circumstances. We will see glands and excretory surfaces, according to the stage of their vital forces, pouring out a host of differing modifications of the same fluid. But what was I saying? They pour out a host of fluids that are really different, for are not the sweat or urine excreted under one circumstance quite different fluids from those excreted under another circumstance? A thousand examples could definitively establish this statement.

By their nature the vital properties become exhausted and in time used up. Heightened in early life, remaining constant in adult life, in later life they become weakened to the vanishing point. It is said that Prometheus, having made some statues of men, stole fire from heaven in order to animate them. This fire is the symbol of the vital properties: as long as it burns, life is supported, only to be annihilated as it gets extinguished. In essence, these vital properties animate matter only for a determinate time, and hence life has necessary limits. Physical properties, on the contrary, are constantly inherent in matter and never leave it. Inert bodies have as a limit to their existence only what chance may assign to them.

Properties independent of life

These are the properties which I consider as pertaining to tissues. Foreign to inert bodies, but inherent in the organs of living bodies, they depend on their texture and the arrangement of their molecules, but not on the life which animates them. Hence, death does not destroy them. They remain in organs which are no longer alive, but nevertheless life increases their energy. Only putrefaction, and the decomposition of organs, destroys them. These properties consist of the extensibility and the tissue contractility which I have discussed in my treatise on life [*Physiological Researches on Life and Death*]. [. . .] I will discuss here a property which has not yet received much attention, which the chemists have noted in their experiments, which the physiologists have most often confused with irritability, but which is as distinct from that as from tissue contractility. I wish to speak of the hardening and contraction through the action of different agents . . . .

Every organized component subjected either postmortem or during life to the action of fire or of certain concentrated acids, contracts and shrivels in various ways and moves almost like irritable organs that are stimulated. We must consider this property under various headings.

(1) Fire is the principal agent for bringing about this hardening. Every living organ placed on burning coals shows this property to the highest degree, in a sudden fashion. (2) Next in order are the very strong acids, first sulfuric, then nitric, then hydrochloric, which make the animal fibres shrivel the most. As the acids get diluted they lose this ability, and the very weak acids do not show it at all. (3) Alcohol, however concentrated it may be, is much less active in producing this effect. Nevertheless, it does shrink little by little the tissues of the parts, condenses them, and even twists them. To preserve anatomical specimens we must dilute the alcohol to approximately a quarter strength. (4) Neutral salts, after taking up the moisture from animal substances, also shrink them and harden them greatly after a certain time. (5) When, by desiccation, the air has removed the aqueous molecules from the solids, these shrivel up and contract in a slow and gradual fashion as the exposure continues. (6) Alkalis,

however strong they may be, never bring about any kind of hardening. (7) Water appears to act in a contrary fashion. Water dilates, expands the organs by maceration, and separates their molecules. Only when a great deal of heat has penetrated does it bring about a hardening. This phenomenon takes place some degrees below that of boiling and is very marked at the boiling point itself.

The different agents of which I have just spoken produce, then, two types of hardening. The first is prompt and sudden, almost like the movement which results from the irritation of a living muscle; the other is slow and gradual, even insensible. Fire and very strong acids act in the first sense. Neutral salts, air, alcohol, and the like, produce predominantly the second.

These two types of hardening differ very much in their result. Where the first type acts, a change soon develops if the hardening agent is not interrupted. Thus, when fire continues to act on solids, it soon ends up by reducing them to a hard and charred mass; boiling water, long continued, destroys little by little the hardened state acquired when the solid organs were plunged into it. A cooking action takes place as the hardness diminishes, and terminates when the solid loses all its consistency and becomes like pulp. In the same fashion the organs of animals which hardened as a result of being plunged in acid, soon grow soft there and change into a real pulp. This double phenomenon produced on the one hand by cooking, on the other hand by strong acids, has the greatest similarity. It seems to derive from the same principle. The difference is that the subsequent softening is much more prompt and is carried out to a greater degree by the second agent than by the first.

The slow and gradual hardening, resulting from contact with neutral salts such as alum, sodium chloride, and the like, represents a phenomenon quite different from the preceding. There is no change into a softened state by the continued action of the active cause. However long this cause acts, it never softens the organ in any slow or gradual fashion. The hardness always remains.

Are these two types of hardening only different degrees of the same principle or do they derive from separate principles? I do not know. I note only that when the living solids have undergone slow and gradual hardening, they are still susceptible to the other type. We know that after several years of desiccation the animal tissues can cornify, just as in the fresh state, by the action of naked fire. I have made the same observation with boiling and with acids. Tissues hardened for a long time in alcohol and in neutral salts present the same phenomenon.

All animal tissues are susceptible to a sudden cornification, except the hair, epidermis and nails which, so to speak, exhibit this in a rudimentary fashion. In general the cornification is more prominent when the organs show a more fibrous character. That is why the muscles, tendons, nerves, and so on, are most susceptible to this change. The non-fibrous organs such as glands and the like show it to a lesser degree. The slow and gradual hardening is virtually the same in all examples. [. . .]

After what we have just said it is clear that solids possess the faculty of contracting or shortening. This faculty can be displayed in several different ways. During life it takes place first by the influence of nerves on voluntary muscles – the 'animal contractility' – and second, in the involuntary muscles, by the action of stimulating agents – the 'sensible organic contractility'. And third, in the muscles, skin, cellular tissue [connective tissue], arteries, veins, and the like, it takes place through the release of stretching. This is the 'tissue contractility' which is lacking or very slight in a great number of organs such as nerves, fibrous bodies, cartilage, bone, and so on. And fourth, it occurs by the action of fire and strong acids. This is the contractility by cornification, and is general.

As soon as life has entirely departed from muscles, they no longer have the first types of contractility, but the third remains, in all organs which possess it. When they are dried up, when they have remained for a while in water, and so on, they lose this also, but the fourth type still remains to them. This is the last to deport from the animal tissues. It remains for many long years. After I had laid bare the cartilagenous parenchyma of bones found in the cemeteries, they were still markedly cornified by fire. I am convinced that this property would be conserved throughout whole centuries, if one could keep the organic tissue this long.

Contractility is, then, a general property, inherent in all animal tissues. But, according to the fashion in which it is manifest, it presents essential differences which divide it into different classes having no analogy one to the other. [. . .]

Of the causes which produce contractility some depend on the existence of life, others are independent thereof and depend only on organization. All organs are essentially contractile, but the causes which make them contract may act only on particular tissues. The hardening alone represents a general effect.

Considerations on the organizations of animals

The properties just analysed are not really inherent in the molecules of matter, but rather disappear as soon as the separate molecules have lost their organic arrangement. The properties belong exclusively to this arrangement, which we must here consider in general fashion.

All animals are an aggregate of different organs which, performing each its own function, cooperate each in its own manner for the conservation of the whole. They are like individual machines in the general machine comprising the individual. These individual machines are in themselves formed by numerous quite different tissues which comprise the true elements of the organs. Chemistry has its simple bodies which, by the various combinations of which they are capable, make up composite bodies – e.g., caloric, light, hydrogen, oxygen, carbon, azote, phosphorous and so on. In the same manner anatomy has its elementary tissues which, by their combinations in various proportions, comprise the organs. These tissues are (1) cellular, (2) the nervous tissue of the animal life, (3) the nervous tissue of the organic life, (4) arterial, (5) venous, (6) exhalant tissues, (7) absorbant tissues and the glands, (8) bony, (9) medullary, (10) cartilagenous, (11) fibrous, (12) fibro-cartilagenous, (13) muscular tissue of the animal life, (14) muscular tissue of the organic life, (15) mucous, (16) serous, (17) synovial, (18) glandular, (19) dermoid, (20) epidermoid and (21) hairy.

These are the real organized elements of our bodily parts. In whatever parts these elements are found, their nature is constantly the same, just as in chemistry the simple (elementary) bodies do not vary, regardless of the compounds they may be forming. [. . .]

[. . .] Simple inspection suffices to show a large number of attributes characteristic of each one and not found in the others.

One has a fibrous character, another glandular, another laminated, still another areolar, and so on. Despite these differences, authors do not agree on the limits of the different tissues. Therefore, to leave no doubt on the point, I have utilized the actions of different reagents. I have examined each tissue and subjected it to the action of heat, air, water, acids, alkalis, neutral salts, and so on. Desiccation, putrefaction, maceration, boiling, and so on, resulting from these different procedures, have changed the character of each tissue in different fashion. We will see that the results have been quite distinct, that in the different alterations each tissue behaves in its own fashion, each gives special products, no two resemble each other. There has been much dispute whether the arterial walls were fleshy, whether the veins had an analogous nature, and so on. If we compare the results from my experiments on different tissues, the question will be at once resolved. It will seem at first that all these experiments have but little result. But I believe they have fulfilled a highly useful goal, of establishing with precision the boundaries of each organized tissue. Since we do not know the real nature of these tissues, we must differentiate them by the different reactions they yield. [. . .]

Since the time of Bordeu, much has been written of the characteristic life of each organ. This is nothing but the specific character which distinguishes the aggregate of vital properties in another. Before these properties had been precisely analysed, it was clearly impossible to form any rigorous idea of this characteristic life. But according to the views which I have just described, wherein most organs are composed of very different simple tissues, the concept of a characteristic life can only be applied to these simple tissues and not to the organs themselves.

Some examples will clarify this important doctrinal point. The stomach is composed of serous, organic muscular, and mucous tissues, and also of all the usual tissues such as the arterial, the venous, and so on, which we can put aside. If you want to envisage in some general way the characteristic life of the stomach, it will be clearly impossible to form any precise or rigorous notion. Actually, the mucous surface is so different from the serous, and both of them so different from the muscular, that to consider them all together is to create confusion. In the same way in the intestines, in the bladder, in the uterus, and so on, if you do not distinguish what pertains to each of the tissues which together make up the organs, the idea of the characteristic life will be only vague and uncertain. [. . .]

Shall I speak of the thoracic organs? What does the life of the fleshy tissue of the heart have in common with that of the membrane which surrounds it? Is the pleura not independent of the pulmonary tissue? Does this tissue have anything in common with the membrane which surrounds the bronchi? I shall ask similar questions about the brain in relation to its membranes, the different parts of the eye, of the ear, and so on.

When we study a function, we must consider in a general fashion the composite organ which performs it; but when we want to know the properties and the life of that organ, we must completely separate it into its elements. In the same way, when you want only general notions of anatomy you can consider each organ as a whole; but if you want to analyse rigorously the intimate structure, it is absolutely necessary to discriminate the tissues.

The conclusions from the preceding principles, relative to disease

[. . .] Since diseases are only the alterations of vital properties, and since each tissue differs from all others in relation to these properties, then clearly each must differ from the others also in its diseases. Thus, in every organ composed of different tissues, one may be diseased, the others remain intact. This is what happens in the great majority of cases. Let us take as an example the principal organs.

(1) Nothing is more rare than the diseases of the cerebral substance; nothing more common than inflammations of the arachnoid which covers it. (2) In the eye most often one membrane alone is diseased, the others preserve their ordinary vitality. (3) In convulsions of the laryngeal muscles or in their paralysis, the mucous surface remains intact; and correspondingly the muscles perform their ordinary functions in catarrhs of this mucous surface. The alterations of either do not affect the cartilages, and conversely. (4) We observe a great many different alterations in the tissue of the pericardium. We almost never find them in the tissue of the heart itself, which is intact when the former is inflamed. The ossification of the membranous lining of the blood vessels does not involve the neighbouring tissues. (5) When the

bronchial mucosa is the seat of a catarrh, the pleura shows but little effect and conversely, in pleurisy the mucosa is not involved. In pneumonia, when in the cadaver an enormous infiltration indicates the tremendous inflammation which has taken place in the pulmonary tissue during life, the serous and mucous surfaces do not often appear to be affected. Those who perform post-mortem examinations know that very often they are intact in early consumption. [. . .]

Since each organized tissue has an arrangement everywhere the same, and since, wherever it is located, it has the same structure and the same properties, quite evidently its diseases must be everywhere the same. Whether the serous tissue belongs to the brain as the arachnoid, to the lung as the pleura, to the heart as the pericardium, to the intestinal viscera as the peritoneum, is a matter of indifference. Everywhere it becomes inflamed in the same manner; everywhere hydropic conditions supervene in a uniform fashion, and so on; everywhere it becomes subject to a sort of eruption of whitish small tubercles, of miliary type, which is, I believe, very little mentioned, but which nevertheless deserves great attention. I have already observed quite a few times this eruption characteristic of the serous tissues, which in general has a chronic course, like the majority of cutaneous eruptions. [. . .] Whatever may be the organ which a mucous tissue covers, its diseases in general have the same character, with variations derived from differences of structure. [. . .]

There are always two classes of symptoms in inflammations: (1) those which bear the nature of the affected tissue; (2) those which depend on the disturbed functions in the organ where it is found. For example, the type of pain, the character of the accompanying fever, the duration, the outcome, and the like, are virtually the same, whatever may be the serous surface that is involved. But if it is the pleura, there is greater difficulty in breathing, a dry cough, and so on; if it is the peritoneum, diarrhoea, constipation, vomiting, and the like; if it is the arachnoid, disturbances of intellectual functions; if the pericardium, an irregular pulse, and so on. The first class of symptoms belongs to every category, the second is more specific and, so to speak, accessory, depending on the proximity of the affected tissue with some other tissue. [. . .]

In conducting these researches we will have to make an important distinction. Certain tissues, such as the bony, the muscular tissue of the animal life, and so on, are exactly the same in all organs where they are found, and consequently their diseases will not differ in any way. Others, such as the cutaneous, the serous, the mucous, and so on, undergo, according to the organs where they belong, certain variations in structure and vital properties which necessarily modify the general phenomena of diseases belonging to these tissues. And finally still others, such as the glandular, the muscular of the organic life, and so on, are very different in each organ. Consequently their general symptoms and their types of diseases must differ greatly. [. . .]

Pierre-Charles-Alexandre Louis

Pierre-Charles-Alexandre Louis (1787–1872) was known as the founder of the *numerical system*, a description clear enough to his contemporaries but one that does not immediately convey to us his particular significance. Louis helped bring about the upsurge in medicine that occurred during the Napoleonic era. The Revolution, when it swept away much of the old tradition, brought to the fore younger men not hampered by established attitudes and methods, and not afraid of innovation. The new growth resulted partly from the urgencies of military medicine, but even more importantly from the initiative of young men who wanted a better understanding of health and disease.

In the late eighteenth century a tide of revolt had been rising against the formalism and rationalism that characterized the Enlightenment. The new movement took different forms. In medicine and science it showed itself in empirical observations and collection of 'facts'. The teachings of Francis Bacon, germinating slowly in the seventeenth century, grew modestly for a century and a half, and then in the late eighteenth century spurted vigorously to flower in the first half of the nineteenth century. The revolutionary and Napoleonic eras in France acted as a powerful force to clear away impediments and permit the new movement to overcome more quickly the restraining forces of tradition. Because of its social and political changes, France could lead the world in medical progress for the first third of the nineteenth century.

In Paris an unrivalled group – men such as Laennec, Bayle, Bichat, Pinel, Corvisart, to name but a few – wrought a profound transformation. And in this group Pierre Louis played an important part.

Born in 1787, he received his medical degree in Paris in 1813 and practised in Russia for seven years. When he realized the inadequacies of his knowledge, he returned to Paris for further study. With single-minded intensity he devoted himself to clinical observations and autopsy dissections in the Paris hospitals.

These hospitals, such as the Charité, the Pitié and the Hotel Dieu, through their great number of patients, made available for study an enormous amount of clinical material. The material was there. Brilliant, hard-working and conscientious physicians made use of it. These men were the glory of French medicine.

Louis immersed himself in a clinical atmosphere and in the post-mortem examinations whereby he could study the anatomical correlates of disease. He tried to approach the patients without preconceptions, but with a mind entirely open to facts. He collected observations, both clinical and anatomical, in an unhurried fashion, and published many important studies, of which the most significant were a book on phthisis in 1825 and another on typhoid in 1829. In 1828 he published journal articles on blood-letting, material that in 1835 appeared in a book. The translation into English (1836) is the source of the present quotations, which include excerpts from the preface, by James Jackson.

Blood-letting had had widespread acceptance, and although some sceptics had denied its validity, the procedure remained a cornerstone of therapeutics. Louis was among those who questioned the validity. Instead of merely theorizing about it, he collected evidence. In his search for precision he sought to reduce his observations to numbers – hence the term 'numerical method'. A quantitative method would allow comparison and, in the presence of adequate controls, would permit valid conclusions. Which variables were important? How could you tell? In his analysis he tried to find relevant new factors or subdivide old ones, and he repeatedly searched for flaws in his own reasoning.

He realized that while no two cases were exactly alike, certain uniformities could be identified, reduced to classes, treated quantitatively and compared. Errors and divergencies arising from individuality will cancel themselves out and could be disregarded. He was thus one of the great pioneers in medical statistics and in clinical research. Even if by our standards his results were halting and imperfect, he nevertheless remains one of the great architects of modern medicine, particularly of modern clinical investigation.

15 Researches on the Effects of Blood-Letting (1836)

Excerpts from P.-C.-A. Louis, *Researches on the Effects of Blood-letting in some Inflammatory Diseases, and on the Influence of Tartarized Antimony and Vesication in Pneumonites*, translated by C. G. Putnam, with Preface and Appendix by James Jackson, Hilliard, Grey & Co., 1836, pp. v–xx, 1–27, 56–65.

Preface by J. Jackson MD

[. . .] If anything may be regarded as settled in the treatment of diseases, it is that blood-letting is useful in the class of diseases called inflammatory; and especially in inflammations of the thoracic viscera. To the general opinion, or belief on this subject, M. Louis gives support by his observations; but the result of these observations is that the benefits derived from bleeding in the diseases, which he has here examined, are not so great and striking, as they have been represented by many teachers.

[. . .]

[. . .]M. Louis has not brought forward a new system of medicine; he has only proposed and pursued a *new method* in prosecuting the study of medicine. This is nothing else than the method of induction, the method of Bacon, so much vaunted and yet so little regarded. But, if so, where is the novelty? If any one, after patiently studying and practising the method proposed by M. Louis, denies the novelty of it, I will not dispute with him a moment. Perhaps he will then agree with me that it is a novelty to pursue the method of Bacon thoroughly and truly in the study of medicine; though it is not new to talk of it and to laud it. [. .].

First, then, he ascertained when the patient under his examination began to be diseased. Not satisfied with vague answers, he went back to the period when the patient enjoyed his usual health; and he also endeavoured to learn whether that usual health had been firm, or in any respect infirm. He noted also the age, occupation, residence and manner of living of the patient; likewise any accidents which had occurred; and which might have influenced the disease then affecting him. He ascertained also, as much as possible, the diseases which had occurred in the family of his patient. Secondly, he inquired into the present disease, ascertaining not only what symptoms had marked its commencement, but those which had been subsequently developed and the order of their occurrence; and recording those, which might not seem to be connected with the principal disease, as well as those which were so connected; also, measuring the degree or violence of each symptom, with as much accuracy as the case would admit. Thirdly, he noted the actual phenomena present at his examination, depending for this not only on the statement of the patient, but on his own senses, his eyes, his ears and his hands. Under this and the preceding head he was not satisfied with noting the functions, in which the patient complained of disorder, but examined carefully as to all the functions, recording their state as being healthy or otherwise, and even noticing the absence of symptoms, which might bear on the diagnosis. Thus all secondary diseases, and those, which accidentally co-existed with the principal malady, were brought under his view. Fourthly, he continued to watch his patient from day to day, carefully recording all the changes, which occurred in him till his restoration to health, or his decease. Fifthly, in the fatal cases he exercised the same scrupulous care in examining the dead, as he had in regard to the living subject. Prepared by a minute acquaintance with anatomy, and familiar with the changes wrought by disease, he looked not only at the parts where the principal disorder was manifested, but at all the organs. His notes did not state opinions, but facts. He recorded in regard to each part, which was not quite healthy in its appearance, the changes in colour, consistence, firmness, thickness, etc.; not contenting himself with saying that a part was inflamed, or was cancerous, or with the use of any general, but indefinite terms.

[. . .]

It was only when he had accumulated a great mass of cases, that M. Louis began to deduce from them any general principles. He then arranged the facts he had collected in a tabular form, so as to facilitate a comparison of them. How much labour this required will be in some measure conceived, when I state that, while going through one class of his observations, those, I believe, which relate to acute diseases, he retired to a distance from Paris and occupied ten months in making out his tables. This statement is, I believe, substantially, if not precisely, correct.

Let the reader conceive of these tables drawn out with accuracy, having columns devoted, with proper discrimination, to each function and to its various derangements, as manifested during life, and to each organ and its lesions as ascertained after death; let him then go to these tables and inquire, under what circumstances certain signs of disease arise, and with what pathological changes in the dead body they are found to correspond; let him ask under what circumstances certain morbid changes of structure occur, and with what symptoms they are found to be connected; he may find the answers and he may obtain them numerically. That is, he may learn in how many cases out of a hundred of any particular disease he will find a certain derangement of a particular function, or a certain change in structure of a particular organ; and he may also learn how often the same things may be noticed in other diseases, with which that under consideration may be compared. [. . .] It is truth only he loves; not anxious to build up a system, nor pretending to explain every thing, he says to his pupils, such and such have been my observations; you can observe as well as I, if you will study the art of observation, and if you will come to it with an honest mind, and be faithful in noting all which you discover, and not merely the things which are interesting at the moment, or those which support a favourite dogma; I state to you the laws of nature as they appear to me; if true, your observations will confirm them; if not true, they will refute them; I shall be content if only the truth be ascertained.

[. . .]

Researches on the effects of blood-letting in some inflammatory diseases [P.-C-.A. Louis]

The results of my researches on the effects of blood-letting in inflammation, are so little in accordance with the general opinion, that it is not without a degree of hesitation I have decided to publish them. [. . .]

These results without doubt will be far from satisfactory; but of what consequence is that, if they are true; since, whatever has this character, cannot fail in the end to be of real utility.

[. . .]

Effect of blood-letting in pleuropneumonia

The cases I am about to investigate are seventy-eight in number; twenty-eight of them proved fatal; and all were in a state of perfect health at the time when the first symptoms were developed.

Of the fifty successful cases, three were bled on the first day of the disease, three on the second, six on the third, eleven on the fourth, six on the fifth, five on the sixth, six on the seventh, as many on the eighth, four on the ninth; [. . .].

But the relation between the length of the disease and the period of the first bleeding, will be made more evident by the following table.

1	2	3	4	5	6	7	8	9
10 3	7 3	19 3	19 3	28 2	13 1	24 2	19 2	35 1
12 2	10 2	29 3	12 2	17 3	16 2	12 4	12 1	11 2
14 2	12 2	20 2	15 2	40 2	23 3	19 2	18 1	17 2
		20	22 4	13 2	35 5	18 2	20 3	30 3
		16 3	12 4	21 2	17 2	15 2	13 2	
		17 4	21 2	13 2		27 2	21 2	
			25 3					
			28 4					
			40 2					
			16 2					
			12 4					
12 2⅓	10 2⅓	20 3	20 3	22 2	21 2⅔	19 2⅓	17 2	23 2

The figures upon the horizontal line above the columns indicate the day when the first bleeding was performed; the figures on the left in each column mark the duration of the disease; those on the right, the number of bleedings; and those on the horizontal line below, show the mean duration of the disease and the average number of bleedings.

That is to say, if it were possible to establish a general proposition from so small a number of facts, it must be concluded that the antiphlogistic treatment, commenced the two first days of a pneumonitis, may very much abridge its duration; whilst after these two days it would make but little difference whether it was commenced a little sooner or a little later. But the amount of difference which exists between these two results, leads us to suspect their exactness; and a thorough examination does in truth show, that the influence of bleeding, when performed within the two first days of the disease, is less than it seems to be at first sight, and that in general its power is very limited.

Indeed – among the cases of the same column in which the antiphlogistic treatment was instituted on the same day, (those of the first and second excepted) the duration of the disease exhibits the greatest variety. Thus in the fourth column, some were convalescent on the twelfth day, others (not to take the extreme) the twenty-fifth and twenty-eighth. This we cannot attribute to the violence of the disease, which was the same; nor to the difference of the treatment, which was equally energetic and directed by the same physician. Whence it seems to result, rigorously, that the utility of bleeding has been very limited in the cases thus far analysed.

Differences no less considerable in the length of the disease would unquestionably have existed among the cases bled within the first twenty-four or forty-eight hours, if their number had been greater. [. . .]

Age had no appreciable influence, everything else being equal, upon the results stated: for this was nearly the same on an average among patients bled for the first time, before the fourth day, and among those who were not bled until after this period; thirty-three years in the first set, and nearly thirty-six in the other.

[. . .]

Perhaps too it will be thought that I have not fixed the exact period of commencement and termination of pneumonitis with sufficient precision, and that its mean duration has been affected by this circumstance. But it seems to me, I have obviated any legitimate objections in this particular, by following in all cases the same method; that is, I have regarded as the commencement of the disease, the period when the patient has experienced a febrile affection, more or less violent, which has been quickly followed or accompanied by pain on one side of the chest and by rusty sputa; these two symptoms appearing at the same time, or nearly the same time; and I have regarded as the time of convalescence the period, at which the sick began to take some light nourishment; three days at least after the febrile action had ceased; although the local symptoms had not disappeared in every case; [. . .].

Finally, the reader will ask, without doubt, whether blood-letting has been the only treatment, of any importance, which has been employed; and in the cases, where other modes of treatment were employed, whether these other modes had not some influence on the mean duration of the disease; or whether they had not counteracted in some degree the good effects of the blood-letting. To this I will answer that vesication was employed in a certain number of cases; but vesication had no appreciable influence on the progress of the disease, as we shall presently see, in the following chapter: so that it will still appear that, in the cases, which we have thus far examined, blood-letting has had but a very limited influence on the course of pneumonitis.

The facts relative to the fatal cases confirm these conclusions, and seem still further to limit the utility of blood-letting. Out of twenty-eight cases in question, eighteen were bled within the four first days of the disease, nine from the fifth to the ninth; [. . .]. This [following] table, which relates to the fatal cases only, shows in each of the columns from left to right, the duration of the disease, the number of bleedings and the ages of the patients; whilst the figure above each column indicates the day when the first bleeding was practised.

1	2	3	4	5	6	7	8	9
6 5 18	53 5 65	4 1 57	29 2 19	16 4 58	62 4 20	20 2 68	25 1 40	22 1 50
	12 3 69	16 2 54	29 4 46	8 2 63	10 2 40			
	8 2 65	6 3 30	12 1 85	9 4 24	29 3 24			
	12 1 55	6 4 47	15 3 37					
	17 7 75	47 2 75	17 1 67					
		11 4 45	20 3 22					
6 5 18	20 3¾ 66	15 3 51	20 2¼ 49	11 3 48	33 3 28	29 2 68	25 1 40	22 1 50

We see, in effect, that the patients who were bled within the four first days of the disease, with the exception of one in the first column, who was eighteen years of age, were older than those who were not actively treated until after this period, in the proportion of fifty-one to forty-three years: this difference may not seem great, but it may have had great influence on the issue of the malady.

[. . .]

From the exposition of facts in this chapter, we infer that blood-letting has had very little influence on the progress of pneumonitis, of erysipelas of the face, and of angina tonsillaris, in the cases under my observation; that its influence has not been more evident in the cases bled copiously and repeatedly, than in those bled only once and to a small amount; that, we do not at once arrest inflammations, as is too often fondly imagined; that, in cases where it appears to be otherwise, it is undoubtedly owing, either to an error in diagnosis, or to the fact that the blood-letting was practised at an advanced period of the disease, when it had nearly run its course; [. . .].

New facts relative to the effect of blood-letting in acute diseases

Since publishing the memoir which forms the subject of the last chapter, I have observed at the hospital of la Pitié, a great number of cases of pneumonitis, of erysipelas of the face, and of angina tonsillaris; and although, in the cases of pneumonitis I have employed blood-letting to the extent of twenty or twenty-five ounces and more, or even to syncope; I have never seen these inflammations arrested in a single case. I believe even that the blood-letting, although usually carried to a greater extent than was practised in the hospital of la Charité, at the time when I made by observations there, has not been more decidedly successful. But these general propositions, founded upon facts trusted, for the most part, to the memory, have too little value to be much regarded; and instead of discoursing, in a vague manner, upon the treatment of forty cases of erysipelas of the face, and one hundred and fifty cases of pneumonitis which have passed under my observation, the last four years, I shall confine myself to giving the reader an analysis of the facts, relative to these two diseases, which I have collected with care during the time of my clinical lectures from 1830 to 1833.

Facts relative to the treatment of pneumonitis

The observations under this head are twenty-nine in number; in four of the cases the disease was fatal; in twenty-five recovery took place, and the patients left the hospital perfectly well.

In all these cases, the patients were in excellent health, when the first symptoms of pneumonitis appeared.

Not a doubt can be entertained as to the character of the disease which affected them, all having expectorated rusty, viscid, semi-transparent sputa; all having had, to a greater, or less extent, crepitous râle, bronchial respiration, and broncophony, with more or less dullness on percussion, in the corresponding part.

Of the twenty-five patients who recovered, no one was bled on the first day of the disease. The first bleeding was on the second, third, fourth, fifth, sixth and seventh days; one case only excepted, that of a patient who was convalescent on the twenty-second day, and who was not bled until the fourteenth. And the disease lasted, on an average, in the order pointed out above, fourteen, eighteen, fourteen, sixteen, nineteen, eighteen and twenty-two days, according to the following table:

2			3			4			5			6			7			14		
15	2	28	11*	2	30	14*	2	32	9*	1	15	25*	1	20	11*	2	34	22*	1	16
16*	3	4	27	2	30	19*	2	24	28*	2	30	21*	1	20	19*	2	37			
11	3	50	28*	2	25	14*	2	27	11	1	20	12*	2	30	18*	2	38			
			9	1	18	12	2	35							24*	1	12			
						13	2	30							21*	2	30			
						15	2	24												
14	2⅔	27	18	1¾	25¾	14	2	29	16	1	21	19	1	23	18	1⅖	30	22	1	16

The ciphers on the first line indicate the days of the first bleeding; those in each column, from left to right, the duration of the disease, the number of bleedings, the quantity of blood drawn. The figures, to which an asterisk is prefixed, also show that the patients to whom they refer, took antimony in large doses.

That is to say, that at the first glance, it would seem rather unimportant whether the patients affected with pneumonitis, were bled, for the first time, on the second, fourth or fifth day of the disease; since its mean duration was nearly the same, in the three lists of cases bled at these different periods. Nevertheless, adding together, on the one side, those who were bled for the first time, from the second to the fourth day inclusive: on the other, those bled afterward; we find the mean duration of the disease to be fifteen days and a half among the first, and eighteen days and a quarter among the second. Hence it would seem fair to conclude that the influence of blood-letting, at a period more or less near to the commencement of the disease, has been a little more marked in the cases now before us, than in those discussed in the first chapter; in which the mean duration of the disease was seventeen days and a half and twenty days.

This difference, although slight, is worthy of remark, especially as it is found in each of the classes of cases, between those who were bled for the first time within the four first days of the disease, and between those who were bled later; which seems to show that it is not accidental.

The difference in the results at the two hospitals is further remarkable, inasmuch as none of the cases, treated at la Pitié, were bled on the first day of the disease; that these patients were, on that account, in a rather less favourable condition than those of la Charité, three of whom were bled on the first day. [. . .]

Examination of the method, followed in the preceding chapters, to determine the therapeutic effects of blood-letting and antimony

[. . .]

The first, and apparently the most weighty objection to the method in question, is that it is difficult to collect a sufficient number of cases of any one disease, which shall be identical; especially if it be remembered that two cases of disease will hardly be found alike in every particular.

Without doubt, if, in order that two cases of the same disease may be classed together, it is considered essential that the individuals should be perfectly equal in age, and mathematically similar in strength, stature and flesh; if the disease must be exactly at the same stage, of the precise extent, (supposing it possible to measure it): if the febrile action must be similar to such a degree, that the pulsations of the arteries in the two cases must not vary two or three strokes; if such are the conditions of the required resemblance, it is impossible that they should ever be found united; any more than that two leaves on the same tree should be found exactly alike in form, colour and thickness. And as there is an evident necessity of uniting similar facts, in order to classify them and draw from them correct conclusions, it would follow that there would be nothing but individualities in medical science; that it would always be impossible to attain any general principle whatever, even in pathology; and also that there would be no means of describing the leaf of a tree in general terms. Experience, fortunately, enables us to appreciate the value of such conclusions, and of the assertion which gives rise to them. A leaf of a tree once well described may always be recognized; and general principles of pathology, once clearly defined, can always be verified under circumstances similar to those, in which the subjects were placed, from whom such general principles were derived. Thus, in truth, we can form a class of facts bearing sufficient resemblance, one to another, and from hence deduce laws which every day's experience verifies.

[. . .]

Let us further remark that the objection made to the numerical method, to wit, the difficulty or impossibility of forming classes of similar facts, is alike applicable to all the methods that might be substituted; *that it is impossible to appreciate each case with mathematical exactness, and it is precisely on this account that enumeration becomes necessary; by so doing, the errors (which are inevitable), being the same in two groups of patients subjected to different treatment, mutually compensate each other, and they may be disregarded without sensibly affecting the exactness of the results.*

[. . .]

The calculus, as I employ it, does not efface differences: *it supposes them*; it limits itself to combining similar unities in order to compare them with parallel unities, these being subjected to somewhat different influences; that if, after all, as has been before remarked, it should sometimes be necessary that facts should be combined, which are not strictly similar; the error will be distributed through the different groups or classes of facts, and will be equalized; so that a comparison can be instituted between several groups without altering the result.

Oliver Wendell Holmes

Puerperal or child-bed fever was one of the truly dread diseases of mankind, which struck sometimes sporadically, sometimes in epidemic form. But although its attacks seemed to be at random, careful observers began to trace out bits of a pattern. Men like Charles White (1728–1813), Thomas Kirkland (1722–98), Alexander Gordon (1752–99) and Robert Collins (1801–96), analysed various aspects of puerperal fever, appreciated its infectious nature, and showed some insight into the ways in which it was spread. They sensed its relation to certain other acute septic states and to putrid substances, filth and overcrowding. They realized that the fever could be controlled, more or less, by appropriate measures directed toward cleanliness.

Oliver Wendell Holmes (1809–94) contributed greatly to the fight against puerperal fever. Holmes, a great figure in American letters, had graduated from Harvard Medical School in 1836 and soon entered an academic career as professor of anatomy. A logical thinker and brilliant writer, he nevertheless had little experience in medical practice. Yet when puerperal fever was arousing particular interest in Boston in the winter of 1842–3, Holmes felt it would be worthwhile 'to learn what experience had to teach in the matter', and he made what is in essence a library study. In 1843 he published a paper in an obscure and short-lived journal, *New England Quarterly Journal of Medicine and Surgery*. The article, brilliant as it is, attracted little attention in the wider community. Later in 1855, at the height of further controversy, it was reprinted, with additions.

Holmes, offering evidence that the physician carried the infection to the obstetrical patient, correlated fresh cases of the disease with particular antecedent activity on the part of the physician, e.g., performing or observing an autopsy on a case of puerperal fever, or attending a patient suffering from the disease. He showed that there was something particularly virulent and highly infectious about the fluids in cases of puerperal fever.

Today, when we know a great deal about streptococci and their role in puerperal fever and erysipelas, Holmes's paper seems a powerful and cogent analysis. Yet without knowledge of the streptococcus the chain of evidence was incomplete and there were discrepancies and contradictions. The new views did not convince the majority of practitioners. Holmes had given us a so-called retrospective study, a form of analysis which has serious pitfalls. And he did not have adequate controls, nor did he measure up to the 'numerical method' which Louis had popularized. Nevertheless the evidence is impressive and the writing is effective.

The most dramatic episode in the fight against puerperal fever revolved around the life of Ignaz Semmelweiss (1818–65) who, ignorant of Holmes's paper, nevertheless came to substantially the same conclusion. Semmelweiss argued not from a survey of the literature but from his own practical experience. Furthermore, he provided concrete statistical evidence in favour of his view. By translating his theories into practice -- by insisting on hand-washing for all those who attended parturient women – he remarkably reduced the mortality from puerperal fever.

He believed that puerperal fever was due to putrid cadaveric material transferred to the pregnant woman. This noxious agent, he believed, was acquired at the autopsy table and conveyed by the examining finger of the physician. Chlorine disinfection of the hands would eliminate the harmful agent. Later, Semmelweiss indicated that the fever might come from putrid matter derived from living organisms, and might find its way through the air. Furthermore, the disease could be transmitted by foul dressings and bed clothes.

Semmelweiss's views, first propounded in 1847, antagonized many powerful physicians. And even fourteen years later, when he published his book on the subject, the opposition remained strong. His own personal tragedy is well known. He showed signs of mental illness, was confined to an asylum in 1865, and soon died from an infection of the finger and arm, presumably a streptococcic cellulitis.

The battle against puerperal infection was won only after considerably more knowledge accumulated and investigators learned a great deal more about bacteria, the mechanisms of infection, and the modes of combating them. Until such knowledge was available, the insight of a few pioneers was not sufficiently cogent to convince the great mass of physicians or laymen.

16 The Contagiousness of Puerperal Fever (1843) [1]

Excerpts from O. W. Holmes, 'The Contagiousness of Puerperal Fever', in *Medical Essays 1842–1882*, Houghton, Mifflin & Co., 1891, pp. 153–69.

I am assured, on unquestionable authority, that 'About three years since, a gentleman in extensive midwifery business, in a neighbouring State, lost in the course of a few weeks eight patients in child-bed, seven of them being undoubted cases of puerperal fever. No other physician of the town lost a single patient of this disease during the same period.' And from what I have heard in conversation with some of our most experienced practitioners, I am inclined to think many cases of the kind might be brought to light by extensive inquiry.

This long catalogue of melancholy histories assumes a still darker aspect when we remember how kindly nature deals with the parturient female, when she is not immersed in the virulent atmosphere of an impure lying-in hospital, or poisoned in her chamber by the unsuspected breath of contagion. From all causes together, not more than four deaths in a thousand births and miscarriages happened in England and Wales during the period embraced by the first report of the Registrar-General. In the second report the mortality was shown to be about five in one thousand. In the Dublin Lying-in Hospital, during the seven years of Dr Collins's mastership, there was one case of puerperal fever to 178 deliveries, or less than six to the thousand, and one death from this disease in 278 cases, or between three and four to the thousand. Yet during this period the disease was endemic in the hospital, and might have gone on to rival the horrors of the pestilence of the Maternité, had not the poison been destroyed by a thorough purification.

[. . .]

In the view of these facts, it does appear a singular coincidence, that one man or woman should have ten, twenty, thirty or seventy cases of this rare disease following his or her footsteps

1. Printed in 1843; reprinted with additions, 1855.

with the keenness of a beagle, through the streets and lanes of a crowded city, while the scores that cross the same paths on the same errands know it only by name. It is a series of similar coincidences which has led us to consider the dagger, the musket and certain innocent-looking white powders as having some little claim to be regarded as dangerous. It is the practical inattention to similar coincidences which has given rise to the unpleasant but but often necessary documents called *indictments*, which has sharpened a form of the cephalotome sometimes employed in the case of adults, and adjusted that modification of the fillet which delivers the world of those who happen to be too much in the way while such striking coincidences are taking place.

I shall now mention a few instances in which the disease appears to have been conveyed by the process of direct inoculation.

Dr Campbell of Edinburgh states that in October 1821, he assisted at the post-mortem examination of a patient who died with puerperal fever. He carried the pelvic viscera in his pocket to the class-room. The same evening he attended a woman in labour without previously changing his clothes; this patient died. The next morning he delivered a woman with the forceps; she died also, and of many others who were seized with the disease within a few weeks, three shared the same fate in succession.

In June 1823, he assisted some of his pupils at the autopsy of a case of puerperal fever. He was unable to wash his hands with proper care, for want of the necessary accommodations. On getting home he found that two patients required his assistance. He went without further ablution, or changing his clothes; both these patients died with puerperal fever. This same Dr Campbell is one of Dr Churchill's authorities against contagion.

Mr Roberton says that in one instance within his knowledge a practitioner passed the catheter for a patient with puerperal fever late in the evening; the same night he attended a lady who had the symptoms of the disease on the second day. In another instance a surgeon was called while in the act of inspecting the body of a woman who had died of this fever, to attend a labour; within forty-eight hours this patient was seized with the fever.

On 16 March 1831, a medical practitioner examined the body of a woman who had died a few days after delivery, from puerperal peritonitis. On the evening of the 17th he delivered a patient, who was seized with puerperal fever on the 19th, and died on the 24th. Between this period and the 6th of April, the same practitioner attended two other patients, both of whom were attacked with the same disease and died.

In the autumn of 1829 a physician was present at the examination of a case of puerperal fever, dissected out the organs, and assisted in sewing up the body. He had scarcely reached home when he was summoned to attend a young lady in labour. In sixteen hours she was attacked with the symptoms of puerperal fever, and narrowly escaped with her life.

In December 1830, a midwife, who had attended two fatal cases of puerperal fever at the British Lying-in Hospital, examined a patient who had just been admitted, to ascertain if labour had commenced. This patient remained two days in the expectation that labour would come on, when she returned home and was then suddenly taken in labour and delivered before she could set out for the hospital. She went on favourably for two days, and was then taken with puerperal fever and died in thirty-six hours.

'A young practitioner, contrary to advice, examined the body of a patient who had died from puerperal fever; there was no epidemic at the time; the case appeared to be purely sporadic. He delivered three other women shortly afterwards; they all died with puerperal fever, the symptoms of which broke out very soon after labour. The patients of his colleague did well, except one, where he assisted to remove some coagula from the uterus; she was attacked in the same manner as those whom he had attended, and died also.' The writer in the *British and Foreign Medical Review*, from whom I quote this statement – and who is no other than Dr Rigby – adds, 'We trust that this fact alone will forever silence such doubts, and stamp the well-merited epithet of "criminal", as above quoted, upon such attempts.'

From the cases given by Mr Ingleby, I select the following. Two gentlemen, after having been engaged in conducting the post-mortem examination of a case of puerperal fever, went in the same dress, each respectively, to a case of midwifery. 'The one patient was seized with the rigor about thirty hours afterwards. The other patient was seized with a rigor the third morning after delivery. *One recovered, one died.*' One of these same gentlemen attended another woman in the same clothes two days after the autopsy referred to. 'The rigor did not take place until the evening of the fifth day from the first visit. *Result fatal.*' These cases belonged to a series of seven, the first of which was thought to have originated in a case of erysipelas. 'Several cases of a mild character followed the foregoing seven, and their nature being now most unequivocal, my friend declined visiting all midwifery cases for a time, and there was no recurrence of the disease.' These cases occurred in 1833. Five of them proved fatal. Mr Ingleby gives another series of seven cases which occurred to a practitioner in 1836, the first of which was also attributed to his having opened several erysipelatous abscesses a short time previously.

I need not refer to the case lately read before this Society, in which a physician went, soon after performing an autopsy of a case of puerperal fever, to a woman in labour, who was seized with the same disease and perished. The forfeit of that error has been already paid.

At a meeting of the Medical and Chirurgical Society before referred to, Dr Merriman related an instance occurring in his own practice, which excites a reasonable suspicion that two lives were sacrificed to a still less dangerous experiment. He was at the examination of a case of puerperal fever at two o'clock in the afternoon. *He took care not to touch the body.* At nine o'clock the same evening he attended a woman in labour; she was so nearly delivered that he had scarcely anything to do. The next morning she had severe rigors, and in forty-eight hours she was a corpse. Her infant had erysipelas and died in two days.

In connection with the facts which have been stated, it seems proper to allude to the dangerous and often fatal effects which have followed from wounds received in the post-mortem examination of patients who have died of puerperal fever. The fact that such wounds are attended with peculiar risk has been long noticed. I find that Chaussier was in the habit of cautioning his students against the danger to which they were exposed in these dissections. The head *pharmacien* of the Hôtel Dieu, in his analysis of the fluid effused in puerperal peritonitis, says that practitioners are convinced of its deleterious qualities, and that it is very dangerous to apply it to the denuded skin. Sir Benjamin Brodie speaks of it as being well known that the inoculation of lymph or pus from the peritoneum of a puerperal patient is often attended with dangerous and even fatal symptoms. Three cases in confirmation of this statement, two of them fatal, have been reported to this Society within a few months.

Of about fifty cases of injuries of this kind, of various degrees of severity, which I have collected from different sources, at least twelve were instances of infection from puerperal peritonitis. Some of the others are so stated as to render it probable that they may have been of the same nature. Five other cases were of peritoneal inflammation; three in males. Three were what was called enteritis, in one instance complicated with erysipelas; but it is well known that this term has been often used to signify inflammation of the peritoneum covering the intestines. On the other hand, no case of typhus or typhoid fever is mentioned as giving rise to dangerous consequences, with the exception of the single instance of an undertaker mentioned by Mr Travers, who seems to have been poisoned by a fluid which exuded from the body. The other accidents were produced by dissection, or some other mode of contact with bodies of patients who had died of various affections. They also differed much in severity, the cases of puerperal origin being among the most formidable and fatal. Now a moment's reflection will show that the number of cases of serious consequences ensuing from the dissection of the bodies of those who had perished of puerperal fever is so vastly disproportioned to the relatively small number of autopsies made in this complaint as compared with typhus or pneumonia (from which last disease not one case of poisoning happened), and still more from all diseases put together, that the conclusion is irresistible that a most fearful morbid poison is often generated in the course of this disease. Whether or not it is *sui generis*, confined to this disease, or produced in some others, as, for instance, erysipelas, I need not stop to inquire.

In connection with this may be taken the following statement of Dr Rigby. 'That the discharges from a patient under puerperal fever are in the highest degree contagious we have abundant evidence in the history of lying-in hospitals. The puerperal abscesses are also contagious, and may be communicated to healthy lying-in women by washing with the same sponge; this fact has been repeatedly proved in the Vienna Hospital; but they are equally communicable to women not pregnant; on more than one occasion the women engaged in washing the soiled bed-linen of the General Lying-in Hospital have been attacked with abscess in the fingers or hands, attended with rapidly spreading inflammation of the cellular tissue.'

Now add to all this the undisputed fact, that within the walls of lying-in hospitals there is often generated a miasm, palpable as the chlorine used to destroy it, tenacious so as in some cases almost to defy extirpation, deadly in some institutions as the plague; which has killed women in a private hospital of London so fast that they were buried two in one coffin to conceal its horrors; which enabled Tonnellé to record two hundred and twenty-two autopsies at the Maternité of Paris; which has led Dr Lee to express his deliberate conviction that the loss of life occasioned by these institutions completely defeats the objects of their founders; and out of this train of cumulative evidence, the multiplied groups of cases clustering about individuals, the deadly results of autopsies, the inoculation by fluids from the living patient, the murderous poison of hospitals – does there not result a conclusion that laughs all sophistry to scorn, and renders all argument an insult?

I have had occasion to mention some instances in which there was an apparent relation between puerperal fever and erysipelas. The length to which this paper has extended does not allow me to enter into the consideration of this most important subject. I will only say, that the evidence appears to me altogether satisfactory that some most fatal series of puerperal fever have been produced by an infection originating in the matter or effluvia of erysipelas.

[. . .]

Of these facts, at the risk of fatiguing repetitions, I have summoned a sufficient number, as I believe, to convince the most incredulous that every attempt to disguise the truth which underlies them all is useless.

There may be some among those whom I address who are disposed to ask the question, 'What course are we to follow in relation to this matter?' The facts are before them, and the answer must be left to their own judgment and conscience. If any should care to know my own conclusions, they are the following; and in taking the liberty to state them very freely and broadly,

I would ask the inquirer to examine them as freely in the light of the evidence which has been laid before him.

1. A physician holding himself in readiness to attend cases of midwifery should never take any active part in the post-mortem examination of cases of puerperal fever.

2. If a physician is present at such autopsies, he should use thorough ablution, change every article of dress, and allow twenty-four hours or more to elapse before attending to any case of midwifery. It may be well to extend the same caution to cases of simple peritonitis.

3. Similar precautions should be taken after the autopsy or surgical treatment of cases of erysipelas, if the physician is obliged to unite such offices with his obstetrical duties, which is in the highest degree inexpedient.

4. On the occurrence of a single case of puerperal fever in his practice, the physician is bound to consider the next female he attends in labour, unless some weeks at least have elapsed, as in danger of being infected by him, and it is his duty to take every precaution to diminish her risk of disease and death.

5. If within a short period two cases of puerperal fever happen close to each other, in the practice of the same physician, the disease not existing or prevailing in the neighborhood, he would do wisely to relinquish his obstetrical practice for at least one month, and endeavor to free himself by every available means from any noxious influence he may carry about with him.

6. The occurrence of three or more closely connected cases, in the practice of one individual, no others existing in the neighbourhood, and no other sufficient cause being alleged for the coincidence, is *prima facie* evidence that he is the vehicle of contagion.

7. It is the duty of the physician to take every precaution that the disease shall not be introduced by nurses or other assistants, by making proper inquiries concerning them, and giving timely warning of every suspected source of danger.

8. Whatever indulgence may be granted to those who have heretofore been the ignorant causes of so much misery, the time

has come when the existence of a *private pestilence* in the sphere of a single physician should be looked upon, not as a misfortune, but a crime and in the knowledge of such occurrences the duties of the practitioner to his profession should give way to his paramount obligations to society.

Samuel Hahnemann

It is much easier to ridicule homoeopathy than to understand it. Hahnemann, the founder of this sect, struggled with important problems, but unfortunately he was poorly equipped to deal with them, so poorly indeed, that his teachings often sound like an utter farrago. The claim that infinitesimal doses of medicines can cure all diseases, or that all chronic ailments are a form of the itch, seem patently absurd. Indeed, great wits from Oliver Wendell Holmes to the present have made fun of homoeopathy. And yet, if we can disentangle the problems that are basic from those that are peripheral, and can shunt aside the maunderings of an old man whose intellect had grown calcified, we can gain rewarding insight into scientific methodology. We can see a strong inner logic, that looked backward rather than forward and ignored 'facts' and the progressive contemporary science.

Samuel Hahnemann (1755–1843) was an anachronism. His ideas were those of the eighteenth century, but they began to attract attention only in the nineteenth century, when the mainstream of progress had already spread far beyond his comprehension. And by this time his personality had become rigid, his mind equally so, and all chance of real progress was lost for him.

In the selections quoted here I have included excerpts of prefatory comments, written by a contemporary disciple of Hahnemann, Constantine Hering. He insisted that homoeopathy be regarded as a branch of natural philosophy, that is, empirical science. Homoeopathy must stand the test of experiment. Theory must depend on fact. These statements have a brave ring and indicate one view of the nature of science, vintage of the 1830s. The remaining excerpts, drawn from Hahnemann's own writings, illustrate the way the complex theory rested on a tenuous foundation, and indicate the gap between assertions of fact and actual empirical verification.

Homoeopathy rests on several interlocking propositions. The first (in a logical rather than chronological sense) defines disease as the assemblage of symptoms from which the patient suffers.

Hahnemann vaguely indicates that symptoms occurred in clusters – a single symptom does not constitute a disease any more than a leg is an entire human body – but he had no concern with real individualized *patterns*. He did not regard diseases as having each a characteristic natural history, but regarded them predominantly as assemblages of symptoms. He was so much against the idea of a disease as a 'thing' or an 'entity' that he failed to provide adequate individualization of diseases.

A second basic postulate: if we eliminate the symptoms, we eliminate the disease. While this may sound merely tautological, it emphasizes the importance of symptomatic treatment as the goal of therapy.

A third principle: medicines – therapeutic agents – produce symptoms. (In more modern terms, we would say that medicines have a demonstrable effect on the body.) But whereas today we would measure physiological or anatomical changes resulting from drug ingestion, Hahnemann regarded only the changes that appeared in consciousness – i.e., 'symptoms'. These symptoms produced by a medication Hahnemann regarded as an 'artificial disease'.

Fourth: the appropriate artificial disease can 'extinguish' the natural disease. The skill of the physician lies in finding the artificial disease that is sufficiently powerful to overcome the naturally occurring ailment.

Now in the context of the late eighteenth century these propositions were by no means absurd. Pharmacology as a scientific discipline did not exist, and there was no systematic investigation of drugs. Hahnemann realized that traditional polypharmacy – the prescribing of multiple drugs at one time for a single condition – could not advance knowledge. The scientific physician had to investigate 'single' drugs, one at a time. But how to do it? Experimental physiology was still but little developed and experimental pharmacology virtually not at all.

Hahnemann was one of the earliest experimental pharmacologists. But he investigated not through physiological and biochemical techniques, which at the turn of the century had not developed to a useful degree, but by introspection, by noting the subjective 'symptoms' that the drugs produced – palpitations, or sweating, or rapid pulse, or dizziness, or nausea, or headache.

A single drug might 'produce' hundreds of different 'symptoms', and all of these had to be carefully noted and codified. The homoeopathic physician then had to select drugs producing symptoms to counteract those of the original disease – i.e., induce an artificial disease that would overcome the original one.

Homoeopathy was a rather curious medical backwater that adopted certain of the forms of scientific medicine and achieved considerable success in its day. It lasted a long time but succumbed as scientific methodology and a critical attitude gradually became more widespread.

17 Organon of Homoeopathic Medicine (1849)

Excerpts from S. Hahnemann, *Organon of Homoeopathic Medicine* (3rd American edn), William Radde (New York), 1849, pp. 14–18, 95–107. [Footnotes are renumbered.]

Preface [Constantine Hering]

Of discoveries

Among men of deliberate and acute reflection, no difference of opinion can exist relative to the truth of a discovery which rests upon the basis of actual experiment. When the author appeals to such experiments, they must be led to a repetition of them, and not oppose their own opinions to the dictates of experience; in fine, they have no other way in forming a judgment than that of accurate and careful experiment.

It may be said that every charlatan, in extolling his nostrums, in like manner appeals to experience, and no one is required for that reason to investigate the merits of his compounds; but it will not be denied that, although the person of the quack may deserve little forbearance, yet the remedy with which he dupes the public may, in some cases, prove beneficial. The old school has received many remedies, mercury among others, from the hands of the quack.

[. . .] None but a vulgar dealer in calumny of the grosser sort, would attempt to degrade Hahnemann to a level with the charlatan; because he promulgates his views and the peculiarities of his method, as a learned physician, and in a manner that is sanctioned by custom, and fully recognised in the history of medicine.

[. . .]

But homoeopathy is not only a new method, but much more. This method does not rest upon new views, like every other hitherto promulgated, but *upon new discoveries, which appertain to the departments of natural philosophy*, the natural sciences, physiology and biology.

The doctrine that every peculiar substance – every mineral, plant, animal, in fact every part of them, or every preparation derived from a preceding one – produces a series of peculiar effects upon the human organism, manifestly belongs to the natural sciences, and only so far to the materia medica as the latter calls these properties into requisition. But it is a science in itself – a science which treats of the effect of a diversity of substances upon the human frame. Whether such a science, in point of fact, be capable of formation, and whether it have any value, can be determined only by experiment. It were equally foolish to deny this without trial, as it was formerly to deny, without exploring, the way which Columbus opened to the west. It would be inexcusable, in the present condition of the *materia medica*, confessedly imperfect, and deficient in all the attributes of a science, to despise this new way of Hahnemann, before knowing, by careful experiment, that it conducts to nothing better.

[. . .]

The cautious investigator will not pass judgment upon all these discoveries, until he shall have performed a series of rigorous experiments. Then only will he be prepared either to reject or accept the method founded thereon, or, at least, learn the useful part of it.

[. . .]

Illustrations

[. . .] Whether the *theories* of Hahnemann are destined to endure a longer or a shorter space, whether they be the best or not, time only can determine; be it as it may, however, *it is a matter of minor importance*. For myself, I am generally considered as a disciple and adherent of Hahnemann, and I do indeed declare, that I am one among the most enthusiastic in doing homage to his greatness; but nevertheless I declare also, that since my first acquaintance with homoeopathy, (in the year 1821) down to the present day, I have never yet accepted a single theory in the *Organon* as it is there promulgated. I feel no aversion to acknowledge this even to the venerable sage himself. It is the genuine Hahnemannean spirit totally to disregard all theories, even those of one's own fabrication, when they are in opposition to the results of pure experience. All theories and hypotheses have no positive weight whatever, only so far as they lead to new experiments, and afford a better survey of the results of those already made.

Organon of medicine [S. Hahnemann]

The sole duty of a physician is to restore health in a mild, prompt, and durable manner.

1. The first and *sole* duty of the physician is to restore health to the sick.[1] This is the true art of healing.

2. The perfection of a cure consists in restoring health in a prompt, mild and permanent manner: in removing and annihilating disease by the shortest, safest, and most certain means, upon principles that are at once plain and intelligible.

[. . .]

In the cure of disease, it is necessary to regard the fundamental cause, and other circumstances

5. When a cure is to be performed, the physician must avail himself of all the particulars he can learn, both respecting the probable *origin* of the acute malady and the most significant points in the history of the chronic disease, to aid him in the discovery of their *fundamental cause*, which is commonly due to some chronic miasm. In all researches of this nature, he must take into consideration the apparent state of the physical constitution of the patient, (particularly when the affection is chronic,) the disposition, occupation, mode of life, habits, social relations, age, sexual functions, etc.

For the physician, the totality of the symptoms alone constitutes the disease

6. The unprejudiced observer, (however great may be his powers of penetration,) aware of the futility of all elaborate speculations that are not confirmed by experience, perceives in

---

1. His mission is not, as many physicians (who wasting their time and powers in the pursuit of fame) have imagined it to be, that of inventing systems by stringing together empty ideas and hypotheses upon the immediate essence of life and the origin of disease in the interior of the human economy; nor is it that of continually endeavouring to account for the morbid phenomena with their nearest cause (which must forever remain concealed) and confounding the whole in unintelligible words and pompous observations which make a deep impression on the minds of the ignorant, while the patients are left to sigh in vain for relief. [. . .]

each individual affection nothing, but changes of the state of the body and mind, (*traces of disease, casualties, symptoms*) that are discoverable by the senses alone – that is to say, deviations from the former sound state of health, which are felt by the patient himself, remarked by the individuals around him, and observed by the physician. The *ensemble* of these available signs represents, in its full extent, the disease itself – that is, they constitute the true and only form of it which the mind is capable of conceiving.[2]

To cure disease, it is merely requisite to remove the entire symptoms, duly regarding, at the same time, the circumstances enumerated in 5

7. As in a disease where no manifest or exciting cause presents itself for removal, (*causa occasionalis*[3]) we can perceive nothing but the symptoms, then must these symptoms alone (with due attention to the accessory circumstances, and the possibility of

2. I cannot, therefore, comprehend how it was possible for physicians, without heeding the symptoms or taking them as a guide in the treatment, to imagine that they ought to search the interior of the human economy (which is inaccessible and concealed from our view), and that they could there alone discover that which was to be cured in disease. I cannot conceive how they could entertain so ridiculous a pretension as that of being able to discover the internal invisible change that had taken place, and restore the same to the order of its normal condition by the aid of medicines, without ever troubling themselves very much about the symptoms, and that they should have regarded such a method as the only means of performing a radical and rational cure. Is not that which manifests itself in disease, by symptoms, identified with the change itself which has taken place in the human economy, and which it is impossible to discover without their aid? Do not the symptoms of disease, which are sensibly cognizable, represent to the physician the disease itself? When he can neither see the spiritual essence, the vital power which produces the disease, nor yet the disease itself, but simply perceive and learn its morbid effects, that he may be able to treat it accordingly? [. . .]

3. It is taken for granted that every intelligent physician will commence by removing this *causa occasionalis*; then the indisposition usually yields of itself. Thus it is necessary to remove flowers from the room when their odours occasion paroxysms of fainting and hysteria, to extract from the eye the foreign substance which occasions ophthalmia; remove the tight

the existence of a miasm) guide the physician in the choice of a fit remedy to combat the disease. The totality of the symptoms, *this image of the immediate essence of the malady reflected externally*, ought to be the principal or sole object by which the latter could make known the medicines it stands in need of – the only agent to determine the choice of a remedy that would be most appropriate. In short, the *ensemble*[4] of the symptoms is the principal and sole object that a physician ought to have in view in every case of disease – the power of his art is to be directed against that alone in order to cure and transform it into health.

When all the symptoms are extinguished, the disease is at the same time internally cured

8. It is not possible to conceive or prove by any experience, after the cure of the whole of the symptoms of a disease, together with all its perceptible changes, that there remains or possibly can remain any other than a healthy state, or that the morbid alteration which has taken place in the interior of the economy has not been annihilated.

[...]

---

bandages from a wounded limb which threatens gangrene, and apply others more suitable; lay bare and tie up a wounded artery where hemorrhage produces fainting; evacuate the berries of belladonna, etc., which may have been swallowed, by vomiting; extract the foreign particles which have introduced themselves into the openings of the body, (the nose, pharynx, ears, urethra, rectum, vagina); grind down a stone in the bladder; open the imperforate anus of the new-born infant, etc.

4. Not knowing at times what plan to adopt in disease, physicians have till now endeavoured to suppress or annihilate some one of the various symptoms which appeared. This method, which is known by the name of the *symptomatic*, has very justly excited universal contempt, not only because no advantage is derived from it, but because it gives rise to many bad consequences. A single existing symptom is no more the disease itself, than a single leg constitutes the entire of the human body. This method is so much the more hurtful in its effects, that in attacking an isolated symptom, they make use solely of an opposite remedy, (that is to say, of antipathics or palliatives) so that after an amendment of short duration, the evil bursts forth again worse than before.

By the extinction of the totality of the symptoms in the process of cure, the suffering of the vital power, that is, the entire morbid affection, inwardly and outwardly, is removed

12. It is solely the morbidly affected vital principle which brings forth diseases,[5] so that the expression of disease, perceptible by the senses, announces at the same time all the internal change, that is, all the morbid perturbations of the vital principle; in short, it displays the entire disease. Consequently, after a cure is effected, the cessation of all morbid expression, and of all sensible changes which are inconsistent with the healthy performance of the functions, necessarily pre-supposes, with an equal degree of certainty, a restoration of the vital principle to its state of integrity and the recovered health of the whole organism.

To presume that disease (non-chirurgical) is a peculiar and distinct something, residing in man, is a conceit which has rendered allopathy so pernicious

13. Disease, therefore, (those forms of it not belonging to manual surgery) considered as it is by the allopathists as *something* separate from the living organism and the vital principle which animates it, as something hidden internally, and material, how subtle soever its nature may be supposed, is a non-entity, which could only be conceived in heads of material mould, and which for ages, hitherto, has given to medicine all those pernicious deviations which constitute it a mischievous art.

Every curable disease is made known to the physician by its symptoms

14. There is no curable malady, nor any invisible morbid change, in the interior of man, which admits of cure, that is not made known by morbid indications or symptoms to the physician of accurate observation – a provision entirely in conformity with the infinite goodness of the all-wise Preserver of men.

5. In what manner the vital principle produces morbid indications in the system, that is, *how* it produces disease, is to the physician a useless question, and therefore will ever remain unanswered. Only that which is necessary for him to know of the disease, and which is fully sufficient for the purpose of cure, has the Lord of life rendered evident to his senses.

*The sufferings of the deranged vital power, and the morbid
symptoms produced thereby, as an invisible whole, one and the
same*

15. The sufferings of the immaterial vital principle which animates the interior of our bodies, when it is morbidly disturbed, and the mass of symptoms produced by it in the organism, which are externally manifested, and represent the actual malady, constitute a whole – they are one and the same. The organism is indeed, the material instrument of life; but without that animation which is derived from the instinctive sensibility and control of the vital principle, its existence is as inconceivable as that of a vital principle without an organism; consequently, both constitute a unit – although, for the sake of ease in comprehension, our minds may separate this unity into two ideas.

[. . .]

*The physician has only to remove the totality of the symptoms,
and he has cured the entire disease*

17. As the cure which is effected by the annihilation of all the symptoms of a disease removes at the same time the internal change upon which the disease is founded – that is to say, destroys it in its totality – it is accordingly clear, that the physician has nothing more to do than destroy the totality of the symptoms in order to effect a simultaneous removal of the internal change – that is, to annihilate the *disease itself*.

[. . .]

*Changes in the general state, in disease, (symptoms of disease)
can be cured in no other way, by medicines, than in so far as the
latter possess the power, likewise, of affecting changes in the
system*

19. As *diseases* are nothing more than *changes in the general state of the human economy* which declare themselves by symptoms, and the cure being impossible except by the *conversion of the diseased state into one of health*, it may be readily conceived that *medicines* could never cure disease if they did not possess the faculty of changing the general state of the system, which

consists of sensation and action, and that their curative virtues are owing to this faculty *alone*.

This faculty which medicines have of producing changes in the system, can only be known by observing their effects upon healthy individuals

20. By a mere effort of the mind we could never discover this innate and hidden *faculty* of medicines – this spiritual *virtue* by which they can modify the state of the human body and even cure disease. It is by experience only, and observation of the effects produced by their influence on the general state of the economy, that we can either discover or form to ourselves any clear conception of it.

The morbid symptoms which medicines produce in healthy persons are the sole indications of their curative virtues in disease

21. [. . .] When medicines act as remedies, they cannot exercise their curative virtue but by the faculty which they possess of modifying the general state of the economy, and giving birth to peculiar symptoms. Consequently, we ought to rely solely upon the morbid appearances which medicines excite in healthy persons, the only possible manifestation of the curative virtues which they possess, in order to learn what malady each of them produces individually, and at the same time what diseases they are capable of curing.

If experience prove that the medicines which produce symptoms similar to those of the disease, are the therapeutic agents that cure it in the most certain and permanent manner, we ought to select these medicines in the cure of the disease. If, on the contrary, it proves that the most certain and permanent cure is obtained by medical substances that produce symptoms directly opposite to those of the disease, then the latter agents ought to be selected for this purpose

22. But, as we can discover nothing to remove in disease in order to change it into health, except the *ensemble* of the symptoms; as we also perceive nothing curative in medicines but their faculty of producing morbid symptoms in persons who are

healthy, and of removing them from those who are diseased, it very naturally follows that medicines assume the character of remedies, and become capable of annihilating disease in no other manner than by exciting particular appearances and symptoms; or to express it more clearly, a certain artificial disease which destroys the previous symptoms – that is to say, the natural disease which they intend to cure. On the other hand, if we wish to destroy the entire symptoms of a disease, we ought to choose a medicine which has a tendency to excite similar or opposite symptoms, according to that which experience may point out to us as the easiest, safest, and most permanent means of removing the symptoms of the disease, and of restoring health, whether it be by opposing to the latter medicinal symptoms that are similar, or contrary.

Morbid symptoms that are inveterate cannot be cured by medicinal symptoms of an opposite character (antipathic method)

23. From pure experience and the most careful experiments that have been tried, we learn that the existing morbid symptoms, far from being effaced or destroyed by contrary medicinal symptoms like those excited by the antipathic, enantiopathic or palliative methods, they, on the contrary, reappear more intense than ever, after having for a short space of time undergone apparent amendment.

The homoeopathic method, or that which employs medicines producing symptoms similar to those of the malady, is the only one of which experience proves the certain efficacy

24. There remains, accordingly, no other method of applying medicines profitably in diseases than the homoeopathic, by means of which we select from all others that medicine (in order to direct it against the entire symptoms of the individual morbid case) whose manner of acting upon persons in health is known, and which has the power of producing an artificial malady the nearest in resemblance to the natural disease before our eyes.

25. Plain experience,[6] an infallible oracle in the art of healing,

6. I do not mean that kind of experience acquired by our ordinary practitioners after having long combated, with a heap of complicated prescrip-

proves to us, in every careful experiment, that the particular medicine whose action upon persons in health produces the greatest number of symptoms resembling those of the disease which it is intended to cure, possesses, also, in reality, (when administered in convenient doses) the power of suppressing, in a radical, prompt, and permanent manner, the totality of these morbid symptoms – that is to say, the whole of the existing disease; it also teaches us that all medicines cure the diseases whose symptoms approach nearest to their own, and that among the latter none admit of exception.

This is grounded upon the therapeutic law of nature, that a weaker dynamic affection in man is permanently extinguished by one that is similar, of greater intensity, yet of a different origin

26. This phenomenon is founded on the natural law of homoeopathy – a law unknown till the present time, although it has on all occasions formed the basis of every visible cure – that is to say, *a dynamic disease in the living economy of man is extinguished in a permanent manner by another that is more powerful, when the latter (without being of the same species) bears a strong resemblance to it in its mode of manifesting itself.*[7]

---

tions, a multitude of diseases which they never examined with care, [. . .]. Fifty years of such experience are like fifty years passed in looking through a kaleidoscope, which, full of unknown things of varied colours, revolves continually upon itself: there would be seen thousands of figures changing their forms every instant without a possibility of accounting for any one of them.

7. Physical and moral diseases are cured in the same manner. Why does the brilliant planet Jupiter disappear in the twilight from the eyes of him who gazes at it? Because a similar but more potent power, the light of breaking day, then acts upon these organs. With what are we in the habit of flattering the olfactory nerves when offended by disagreeable odours? With snuff, which affects the nose in a similar manner, but more powerfully. Neither music nor confectionary will overcome the disgust of smelling, because these objects have affinity with the nerves of other senses. By what means does the soldier cunningly remove from the ears of the compassionate spectator the cries of him who runs the gauntlet? By the piercing tones of the fife, coupled with the noise of the drum. By what means do they drown the distant roar of the enemy's cannon, which carries terror to the heart of the soldier? By the deep-mouthed clamour of the big drum. Neither the

The curative virtues of medicines depend solely upon the resemblance that their symptoms bear to those of the disease

27. The curative powers of medicines are therefore grounded upon the faculty which they possess of creating symptoms similar to those of the disease itself, but which are of a more intense nature. It necessarily follows, that disease cannot be destroyed or cured in a certain, radical, prompt and permanent manner, but by the aid of a medicine which is capable of exciting the entire group of symptoms which bear the closest resemblance to those of the disease, but which possess a still greater degree of energy.

Some explanation of this therapeutic law of nature

[. . .]

29. Every disease (which does not belong exclusively to surgery) being a purely dynamic and peculiar change of the vital powers in regard to the manner in which they accomplish sensation and action, a change that expresses itself by symptoms which are perceptible to the senses, it therefore follows, that the homoeopathic medicinal agent, selected by a skilful physician, will convert it into another medicinal disease which is analogous, but rather more intense.[8] By this means, the natural morbific

---

compassion nor the terror could be suppressed by reprimands or a distribution of brilliant uniforms. In the same manner, mourning and sadness are extinguished in the soul when the news reach us (even though they were false) of a still greater misfortune occurring to another. The evils resulting from an excess of joy are mitigated by coffee, which, of itself, disposes the mind to impressions that are happy. The Germans, a nation which had for centuries been plunged in apathy and slavery by their princes – it was not till after they had been bowed to the dust by the tyranny of the French invader, that a sentiment of the dignity of man could be awakened within them, or that they could once more arise from their abject condition.

8. [. . .] Natural diseases, simply because of their more tedious and burthensome operation (as psora, syphilis, sycosis), cannot be overcome or extinguished by the unaided vital energies, until these are more strongly aroused by the physician, through the medium of a very similar yet more powerful morbific agent (a homoeopathic medicine). Such an agent, upon its administration, urges, as it were, the insensate, indistinctive vital energies, and is substituted for the natural morbid affection hitherto existing. The vital energies now become affected by the medicine alone, yet transiently; because its effect (that is to say, the natural course of the medicinal disease thereby excited) is of short duration.

power which had previously existed, and which was nothing more than a dynamic power without substance, terminates, while the medicinal disease which usurps its place being of such a nature as to be easily subdued by the vital powers, is likewise extinguished in its turn, leaving in its primitive state of integrity and health the essence or substance which animates and preserves the body.

Part Four **Fruition**

Rudolf Virchow

Rudolf Virchow (1821–1902) lived at the 'right' time. A man of great talent, he grew to maturity in a period of transition and intellectual unrest, and his very energy and ability helped to shape that transition and direct medical science into remarkably productive channels.

In the first third of the nineteenth century France easily led the medical world, while in Germany medicine was at a low ebb. The empirical approach of the great French clinicians, and their concern with the natural history of disease, contrasted sharply with the philosophic system-making of German *Naturphilosophie*.

Several major trends converged, so to speak, and rendered possible the steady climb of German medicine to a position of dominance. First was a spirit of rebellion. Younger men of great talent, growing up after the Napoleonic era, rebelled against the established medical hierarchy, and wanted to get into the mainstream of science. A great upsurge in physiology and biochemistry opened up new viewpoints to the medical investigator, particularly with the concepts of *process*, of dynamic activity and interaction. Then, in the 1830s the microscope became a powerful tool for critical investigation. Advances in optics and technology permitted more precise and reliable observation. Improved microscopy led to the cell theory, which quite transformed biological thinking.

Rudolf Virchow grew up in this period, exciting enough in science, even more exciting in social and political activities. Born in 1821, he studied medicine in Berlin and received his MD degree in 1843. He had a strong experimental bent, and early in his career became an excellent microscopist. He was ambitious, aggressive and rebellious, and also endowed with great self-confidence. One of his early triumphs was his attack on the leading pathologist of the era, Rokitansky, who held humoralist views quite inconsistent with the newest teachings in biology.

Virchow held advanced sociological views. The Prussian government had sent him to investigate a typhus epidemic in

Silesia: in his report he not only discussed the medical situation but also emphasized the need for democracy, education, freedom and prosperity in the community, as important aspects for preventing epidemics. His liberal social views prompted him even to fight on the barricades in Berlin, in 1848.

He left Berlin for Würzberg, to become professor of pathologic anatomy, the first chair of its kind ever to be established. His excellent work resulted in his being recalled to Berlin in 1856. From this vantage point he influenced the entire realm of western medicine.

When he was only twenty-six years old, he founded the *Archiv für pathologische Anatomie und Physiologie*, which became one of the leading scientific periodicals in the world. In addition to his work in pathology, he achieved prominence in anthropology and archaeology. Furthermore, he mingled in practical politics, served in the Prussian lower house for many years and sat in the Reichstag from 1880 to 1893, as an opponent of Bismarck.

He is famous for his insistence that all cells derive from pre-existing cells, the *omnis cellula a cellula* – not original with him but owing its popularization largely to his efforts. Later he expounded quite erroneous views about the nature of carcinoma, and had little sympathy for the new discoveries in bacteriology or for the teachings of evolution. His great reputation and widespread influence, together with his dogmatism, made his errors all the more pernicious.

The selections I have chosen here come in part from his essay of 1847, discussing the scientific viewpoint of medicine, and in part from a follow-up article written thirty years later. These quotations show one of Virchow's prevailing faults, a windy rhetoric that reflects the philosophic heritage he tried to escape. Nevertheless he does propound a point of view that is crucial for medical thought. He emphasized the biological character of medicine and the proper methodology, and made clear that mere anatomical observation represents only a part of the broader view of truly scientific medicine. Despite all his arrogant dogmatism the message he tried to give has relevance for physicians at all times. While his essay started out with concern for German medicine, he discussed problems of medical research, practice and attitudes that will repay careful thought today.

18 Standpoints in Scientific Medicine (1847)

Excerpts from R. Virchow, 'Standpoints in Scientific Medicine (1847)' in *Disease, Life and Man: Selected Essays*, translated by Lelland J. Rather, Stanford University Press, 1958, pp. 26–39.

When we speak of scientific medicine, at the present time, it is highly necessary to reach agreement among ourselves concerning the meaning of the words.

According to our point of view it is self-evident that medicine involves the art of healing – although the most recent developments in medicine may make it appear as if this had hardly anything to do with the matter. Only those who regard healing as the ultimate goal of their efforts can, therefore, be designated as physicians.

Ever since we recognized that diseases are neither self-subsistent, circumscribed, autonomous organisms, nor entities which have forced their way into the body, nor parasites rooted on it, but that they represent only the course of physiological phenomena under altered conditions – ever since this time the goal of therapy has had to be the maintenance or the re-establishment of normal physiological conditions.

The actual accomplishment or, put more precisely, the striving for an actual accomplishment, of this aim comprises the task of practical medicine.

Scientific medicine, for its part, has as its object the investigation of those altered conditions which characterize the diseased body or various ailing organs, the identification of abnormalities in the phenomena of life as they occur under specifically altered conditions, and, finally, the discovery of means for abolishing these abnormal conditions. It presupposes therefore a knowledge of the normal course of the phenomena of life and the conditions under which this course is possible. It is therefore based on physiology. Scientific medicine is compounded of two integrated parts – pathology, which delivers, or is supposed to deliver, information about altered conditions and altered physiological phenomena, and therapy, which seeks out the means of restoring or maintaining normal conditions.

Thus practical medicine is never the same thing as scientific medicine but rather, even in the hands of the greatest master, an application of it. The scientific practitioner, however, distinguishes himself from the *routinier* and the medical opportunist by making the achievements of scientific medicine his own, so that they form the basis of his performance and he serves neither the idol of accustomed routine nor that of chance.

Medicine presents itself to us in this aspect if we project an ideal picture of it. Let us not deceive ourselves into believing that the realization of this picture is not still far in the future. We know only in a very fragmentary fashion the conditions which determine the appearance of abnormal phenomena in the living organism, and even when we do know these conditions, often enough we do not, to our regret, know the means to eliminate them. Under such circumstances the practical physician has the right to cherish a certain degree of empiricism, but so much the greater is his obligation to abolish this empiricism by means of his own observations and to help in the raising of the glorious structure of scientific medicine. The clinical physician is chiefly obligated because the clinic is the focus of medical practice. Hence the control of a clinic is such an extremely important matter at the present time, since the clinician of our day must be not only a scientific practitioner but an observer and investigator as well.

It is said that there are circumstances in which the split between scientific and practical medicine is so great that the learned physician can do nothing, while the practical physician knows nothing. Lord Bacon has said, *scientia est potentia*. Knowledge which is unable to support action is not genuine – and how unsure is activity without understanding! [. . .] In Germany, at the time of the revolution, a philosophy was born, a philosophy which turned itself further and further away from nature, and a return to nature was possible only after this philosophy brought about its own dissolution. This return to nature manifested itself in the history of medicine in three stages: the stages of nature-philosophy, of natural history, and lastly, of natural science. Everyone knows the principles by which these three points of view have influenced medicine. The significance of each stage may best be assessed from the position which each assigns to hypothesis, since the three stages are characterized by a transition from an easygoing procedure to one less so, and culminate finally in a strict method. The school of the nature-philosophers, as is well known, based its medical system on its philosophy; to it logical hypothesizing was a completely justifiable equivalent for observation. The school which followed, calling itself very accurately the 'natural-historical', partly absorbed this point of view during its development, and specifically it elevated proof by analogy to a position of extreme importance, exploiting everything from the whole of nature as it was understood, including past and present medical knowledge, and, with a great deal of spirit, erecting a structure whose supporting pillars were so many analogies and hypotheses. Medicine later reached the natural-scientific stage at a time when philosophy, too, had begun to turn itself toward nature and life; just as philosophy vindicated the old rights of the senses, so medicine threw off belief, cashiered the authorities, and relegated hypotheses to a housebroken existence. While used frequently enough in private, they are left at home when we step into the public forum. Both medicine and philosophy are in agreement that only a serious study of life and its phenomena can assure for them a place of significance. Only a precise understanding of the conditions of individual and community life will make it possible to establish the laws of medicine and philosophy as general laws of mankind, and only then will the saying *scientia est potentia* be fulfilled.

[. . .]

It must be realized that now is not the time for systems, but the time for detail-investigations. There is a certain danger of a retrogression to crude empiricism in this procedure, but the danger is present only so long as an arbitrary attempt is made to draw general conclusions from detail-investigations. This is an error which the 'systematic spirit of the Germans' has committed often enough; and it will disappear to the extent that the number of investigators, and hence the number of detail-investigations, increases. Let us seek general laws in the sum of these specific phenomena, but let us refrain from constructing systems which derive the phenomena from *a priori* general laws, or general laws from isolated phenomena. We have no use for systems until our experience is sufficiently inclusive to give us the guarantee that the system contains truth.

Chemistry has already accomplished a great deal for us, although thus far very little is useful for practical purposes. We expect a great deal more from it, but only if it devotes itself to individual phenomena more often, and places itself in the position of spokesman for medicine less often, than heretofore. We can learn much from chemistry, but we will have to reserve for ourselves the privilege of applying its findings.

General and developmental anatomy have given us much information about individual phenomena, but they can never give us a comprehension of the conditions determining these phenomena. These sciences, therefore, can never and will never participate in the real kernel of medicine, the art of healing. Pathology as well as therapy can be constructed only from within outward, and we dispute the right of any discipline not itself rooted in the contemplation of diseased life to share in the interpretation of its phenomena.

In this connection it appears to me that all those who understand the situation agree that pathological anatomy is the anteroom of medicine, and it would please me, least of all, to detract from its value. However, in the interest of pathological anatomy itself it appears to me advisable to elaborate on the value and significance of the subject for medicine, and to puncture certain extravagant hopes which have been founded on this discipline.

Often enough one hears the reproach that pathological anatomy has to do with end-stages but not with disease itself. Those who say this are half right and half wrong. It would amount to closing one's eyes before the facts of nature to deny that almost all diseases bring forth material, sense-perceptible changes in the body which of necessity belong to the history of the disease, and that the majority of diseases are accompanied from the beginning on by highly decisive, pathognomonic, material disturbances. To this extent, it is incorrect to doubt the significance of pathological anatomy in medical science. However, pathological anatomy has another side, and when this is considered, its opponents have a good deal of justification.

Let us consider for a moment the natural sciences in general, with respect to the mechanics of their development. Every natural science begins with a description of individual objects, more or less rapidly followed by their classification, to which, finally, the story of the origin and development of these objects is added. The descriptive part is only propaedutic and its greatest achievements can have no more than an aesthetic interest; it is thus that we learn to know the properties of things, without learning of their interrelationships. Classification is a requirement of the ordering intellect; though it can be scientific to a high degree, its significance is nevertheless purely practical; it is used for scientific orientation and mutual, effortless communication. Genuine science commences with the history of material bodies; it inquires into the mechanisms and circumstances of their origin and development, into the temporal and causal interrelationships between these bodies, being concerned less with bodies as such than with processes in them, that is, with phenomena and motion. This part of science can in general be designated physiological; the first two parts, anatomical.

Now in what manner does the scientific investigator build up the physiological part? Let us take one example. It had been known for a long time that all bodies possessed, to a certain degree, the property of heaviness; thus this was a general law. Newton saw an apple fall to the earth from a tree in consequence of this heaviness, and he asked himself why the apple did not fall toward the sky. Investigating this question further, he discovered the new law that bodies were attracted along radii directed toward the centre of the earth. Turning his attention to the heavens and seeing the phenomena of the earth repeated there on a grand scale, he discovered the still higher law describing the mutual attraction of the heavenly bodies – a law which has recently been confirmed, in one of the greatest triumphs of human assiduity, by the discovery of a new planet. Newton went further, however, and formulated a hypothesis which he could not prove, since the available facts were not sufficient for this, the hypothesis of the existence of a mutual attraction between all matter. This hypothesis, a generalization of a proven law and a rational consequence of this law, was itself elevated to the position of a law by the reflections of the following centuries.

Scientific investigation proceeds therefore in the following manner: a phenomenon of general occurrence is elevated to the position of a law, and when this law is applied to things which have not yet been discovered, a hypothesis is set up. Evidence is gathered for the proof – or better, for the testing – of this hypothesis in order to find a new law. Hypothesis is thus an essential part of scientific investigation, for it represents the thinking which must precede every rational action. To an equal degree analogy belongs to scientific investigation, for it is precisely by the drawing of analogies that the generalization of a known law to form a new hypothesis is carried out. The hypotheses and analogies in themselves have no value in scientific investigation except to the extent that they function as entering wedges for further investigation. The interest which our hypotheses have for us is thereby explained, for they are the growing and developing laws on which we test our strength, while the already discovered and firmly established facts belong to a past which every moment makes more alien to us.

[. . .]

Pathological anatomy in large part owes the great importance which it has assumed in modern times to ignorance, specifically to a complete lack of acquaintance with its history. [. . .] There is no longer a place for pathological anatomy as a dogmatic science; everyone must be clearly aware of the proofs for each law. But where to obtain proofs if the whole argument begins with a hypothesis? [. . .] I will limit myself to the conclusion that pathological anatomy is really an anatomical science, not a physiological one, and that it can therefore make decisions concerning purely anatomical questions with the greatest of security, but concerning physiological questions only with great insecurity. Objects which we see only in their spatial relationships are supposed to be brought into a temporal and causal relationship. Is pathological anatomy able to do this in a precise scientific manner? In some instances, far more often than appears at first sight when the approach is made in a sufficiently unprejudiced manner, certainly; very frequently not at all. Although the most empirical and casuistic of all sciences, pathological anatomy as practised up to the present time can only become a modern panegyrist of hypothesis. For how can one decide with certainty which of two coexistent phenomena is the cause and which the effect, whether one of them is the cause at all instead of both being effects of a third cause, or even whether both are effects of two entirely unrelated causes?

The final decision in these matters belongs to a science which at the present time exists only in rudiments and which appears destined to replace general pathology; I refer to pathological physiology. We define pathological physiology as the essential theoretical part of scientific medicine. 'Theoretical' is obviously not the same as 'hypothetical' since the former starts from observation and the latter from arbitrary decision. Pathological anatomy is the doctrine of deranged structure; pathological physiology is the doctrine of deranged function. It includes, therefore, pathological changes of the blood, the phenomena of abnormal circulation, respiration, nutrition and secretion, the study of exudation and the metamorphoses which occur in it – in other words, the development of pathological processes – and finally, the study of altered muscle and nerve activity. It might seem as if all of this were very simple, as if one had merely to write out the laws of ordinary physiology and apply them to the several pathological processes. If physiology were complete, this might perhaps be correct; however, physiology, though a 'respectable' science, is thus far a very incomplete one. When one asks detailed questions, one receives, often enough, a Delphic answer only. Physiology is not entirely responsible for this, since the detailed questions have hardly yet been placed before her by pathology.

What remains now to be done? The most comfortable and well-trodden way is to pass over such places with the aid of flying bridges of hypothesis and analogy. But if somebody follows behind with a more heavily laden wagon, the flimsy bridges collapse (if, indeed, they are still standing) and a state of sorry perplexity overcomes the leaders. It is for this reason that a pathological physiology is necessary, a physiology which does not stand before the gates of medicine but lives in its mansion, a science which knows exactly what medicine lacks, what investigations are required, and what questions need to be answered. Pathological physiology receives its questions in part from pathological anatomy, in part from practical medicine; it derives its answers partly from observation by the sickbed, to this extent being a division of the clinic, and partly from animal experiment Experiment is the final and highest court of pathological physiology, for experiment alone is equally accessible to the entire world of medicine, and experiment alone shows the specific phenomenon in its dependency on specific conditions, for these conditions are arranged by choice.

[. . .]

Once again, therefore, let us not deceive ourselves about the present state of medicine! It is undeniable that our spirits are exhausted by the innumerable hypothetical systems which are constantly being thrown to the winds and replaced by new ones. A few more mishaps, however, and this time of disturbance will have passed by and it will be understood that only calm, industrious, and steady work, true work of observation or experiment, has permanent value. Pathological physiology will then gradually reach full fruition, not as the creation of a few overheated heads, but from the cooperation of many painstaking investigators; a pathological physiology which will be the stronghold of scientific medicine, where pathological anatomy and the clinic are only the outworks!

19 Standpoints in Scientific Medicine (1877)

Excerpts from R. Virchow, 'Standpoints in Scientific Medicine (1877)' in *Disease, Life and Man: Selected Essays*, translated by Lelland J. Rather, Stanford University Press, 1958, pp. 142–9.

It was just thirty years ago, in April 1847, that under this same title I wrote the first paper for the initial issue of these Archives. Now, as we begin the seventeenth volume, if I recall a time lying so far in the past, I do so with the wish that the younger generation now beginning to contribute to the progress of science may look back with us at the goals which their elders set up a generation ago and have since unwaveringly pursued.

At that time we attempted to shake off the spell which philosophy, nature-philosophy in particular, had for a long period cast over science. We fought against *a priori* speculation; we rejected systems, and we relied solely on experience. It was not long before we were reproached for contributing to the decline of science, for putting an endless array of bare and detailed facts in the place of ordered knowledge, and for ruthlessly sacrificing millennia of practice on the altar of natural science without offering the helpless beginner a firm basis for his actions.

We did not permit ourselves to be frightened by either the number or the stature of our opponents. Undisturbed, we confined ourselves to the investigation of isolated problems, completely confident that every new fact would necessarily spread light in fields as yet dark, and that every forward step would to some extent increase our insight into the sequence of natural events and thereby broaden our view of natural processes. And we were not deceived. The medicine of today so little resembles the medicine of that time, and differs so greatly from two thousand years of traditional medicine, that it is already considered an indication of special erudition today when someone still commands a full and unprejudiced understanding of the past. How few among physicians of the present day are able to place themselves in the spirit of an era which did not yet know that capillaries are real vessels with definite walls, that organic muscle fibers are the bearers of movement even in the smallest organoid formations of the body, and that the delicacy of the peripheral nerve network exceeds even the boldest speculations! Yes, how few suspect that the period when all of this was unknown lies only thirty years behind us! What an effort it has cost to overturn a system of humoral pathology secured by a thousand bonds of language and popular tradition, and to set up in its place a straightforward science based on direct experience with a realistic view of the tissues and their significance for pathology and therapy! What efforts had to be made, what ever-renewed and minute investigations, in order to introduce the genetic principle into pathology, to establish the developmental history of individual processes, and to assign every phenomenon, whether it belonged to the progressive or regressive, the active or passive, the nutritive, formative, or functional category, to its proper place! And yet we have succeeded in bringing firm order out of seeming chaos; the thousands of individual facts have been comprehended in a few well-established laws and made easily accessible to the understanding of the younger generation in this new order.

[. . .]

We were enemies of philosophy, to be sure, but not of philosophy in general, only of the cocksure, all-knowing, self-satisfied philosophy of the forties. We did not find our method – the currently accepted scientific method – without philosophy. We had respect not only for the 'logic of facts', but for logic in general; we exerted ourselves to take up the old well-founded and thoroughly worked out logic, rather than to adjust our standard to the demands of a self-developed logic new for each special case. We were not blind to the advantages of dialectic. We sought for clear-cut conceptions, precision of expression, and correct terminology. We exerted ourselves to introduce a scientific language into medicine and to put our newly won understanding beyond the reach of wanton distortion, whether by impressions of the moment, by improper generalization, or by the tendency to the figurative misuse of conceptions.

[. . .]

It is no longer necessary today to write that scientific medicine is also the best foundation for medical practice. It is sufficient to point out how completely even the external character of medical practice has changed in the last thirty years. Scientific methods have been introduced everywhere into practice. The diagnosis and prognosis of the physician are based on the experience of the pathological anatomist and the physiologist. Therapeutic doctine has become biological and thereby experimental science. Concepts of healing processes are no longer separated from those of physiological regulatory processes. Even surgical practice has been altered to its foundations, not by the empiricism of war, but in a much more radical manner by means of a completely theoretically constructed therapy.

Claude Bernard

Claude Bernard (1813–78) belonged to the post-Napoleonic generation and consequently he enjoyed the benefits which the revolutionary period and the Napoleonic aftermath wrought in French medicine. The latter eighteenth century and the first quarter of the nineteenth century witnessed a new empiricism and a new scientific attitude, which permeated both the clinic and the laboratory. Among clinicians Laennec (1781–1826), discoverer of the stethoscope, epitomized this scientific spirit, involving as it did a respect for facts, concern with discovering new data and caution in making generalizations. Magendie (1783–1855), who followed Laennec as professor of medicine at the University of Paris, achieved his greatest fame as a physiologist. Claude Bernard studied under Magendie, and eventually succeeded him as professor of medicine. Bernard was entirely an experimentalist who never practised medicine, yet he influenced the entire methodology of medicine and helped to make both the clinic and the laboratory more truly scientific.

Claude Bernard began his career by serving a brief apprenticeship to a local pharmacist (1832–3), but he heartily disliked the profession preferring literature and play-writing. He secured a release from his apprenticeship after serving only eighteen months and then, at the age of twenty, he set off for Paris with a stage play in his pocket. Although his manuscript met a cool reception, he did receive some good advice, that he study medicine as a means of livelihood while he continued his writing.

But medicine proved a greater lure. Under the influence of Magendie, he devoted himself to physiology. At first, professional advancement was difficult. He was unsuccessful in competition for academic posts and he had a serious financial struggle. But he was a prodigious worker, a keen observer, and an excellent experimentalist. With his researches on the function of the pancreatic juice (1846–9) he achieved his first great success.

His work developed out of 'chance observations' on rabbit urine. Ordinarily rabbit urine is alkaline and turbid, as in herbivores. When Bernard noted clear acid urine, characteristic of carnivores, the idea occurred to him that the rabbits, when in transit, had been fasting and actually living on their own flesh. He devised experiments to test his hypothesis, and in the course of these, his attention was drawn to the lacteals, and then to the pancreas and its role in the digestion of fats. His observations gave rise to ideas which he tested experimentally. He grasped the implications of what he saw and did; he provided chains of reasoning and experimentation, to achieve an understanding of recondite physiological functions.

After this success, recognition was rapid. He was elected to the Academy of Sciences in 1854, and on the death of Magendie, to the chair of medicine.

His experimental researches ranged widely. Apart from the studies on the pancreas his major contributions include his work on curare, on the vasomotor control of the circulation and, above all, on carbohydrate metabolism, especially the role played by the liver. He devised the term 'internal secretion' and introduced the concept of 'internal environment' that forms such an important part of physiological thinking.

Bernard stands in contrast to Xavier Bichat who, as a vitalist, insisted on the fundamental distinctions between the living and the non-living. Bichat stressed the inconstancy as evidence that living beings obeyed laws quite distinct from physics and chemistry. Bernard, on the other hand, strongly opposed vitalism. He insisted that biological phenomena, if suitably studied, were as regular as those of physics and chemistry and, moreover, obeyed the same laws. This he could demonstrate in his own work, for the physiologist can set rigid conditions for his experiments, introduce strict controls, and demonstrate reproducible uniformities. The clinician has much greater difficulty but nevertheless, as we have seen with Louis, can make progress in this direction.

Claude Bernard's greatest work and the one from which we quote here, was the *Introduction to the Study of Experimental Medicine* (1865) in which he discussed and illustrated the proper methodology in science, particularly medicine. Although the subject had long engaged philosophers, and many physicians had much to say on the topic, Bernard brought a new clarity and cogency that was particularly influential.

20 An Introduction to the Study of Experimental Medicine (1865)

Excerpts from C. Bernard, *An Introduction to the Study of Experimental Medicine*, translated by Henry Copley Green, Dover Publications, 1957, pp. 2–21.

Scientific medicine, like the other sciences, can be established only by experimental means, i.e., by direct and rigorous application of reasoning to the facts furnished us by observation and experiment. Considered in itself, the experimental method is nothing but reasoning by whose help we methodically submit our ideas to experience – the experience of facts. [. . .]

Reasoning is always the same, whether in the sciences that study living beings or in those concerned with inorganic bodies. But each kind of science presents different phenomena and complexities and difficulties of investigation peculiarly its own.

Reasoning will always be correct when applied to accurate notions and precise facts; but it can lead only to error when the notions or facts on which it rests were originally tainted with error or inaccuracy. That is why experimentation, or the art of securing rigorous and well-defined experiments, is the practical basis and, in a way, the executive branch of the experimental method as applied to medicine.

[. . .] By simply noting facts, we can never succeed in establishing a science. Pile up facts or observations as we may, we shall be none the wiser. To learn, we must necessarily reason about what we have observed, compare the facts and judge them by other facts used as controls. But one observation may serve as control for another observation, so that a science of observation is simply a science made up of observations, i.e., a science in which we reason about facts observed in their natural state, as we have already defined them. An experimental science, or science of experimentation, is a science made up of experiments, i.e., one in which we reason on experimental facts found in conditions created and determined by the experimenter himself.

Certain sciences, like astronomy, will always remain sciences of observation, because the phenomena studied are outside our sphere of action; but terrestrial sciences may be, at once, sciences of observation and experimental sciences. Let me add that all these sciences begin as sciences of pure observation; only as we go into the analysis of phenomena do they become experimental, because the observer, turning experimenter, invents methods of investigation to penetrate bodies and vary the conditions of phenomena. Experimentation is only utilizing methods of investigation peculiar to experimenters.

Now experimental reasoning is absolutely the same, whether in sciences of observation or in experimental sciences. We find the same judgment by comparison based on two facts, one used as starting point, the other as conclusion, of our reasoning. Only in the sciences of observation, the two facts are always observations; while in the experimental sciences, the two facts may be taken exclusively from experimentation, or at the same time from experimentation and from observation, according to the special case and according to how deeply we go into experimental analysis. A physician observing a disease in different circumstances, reasoning about the influence of these circumstances, and deducing consequences which are controlled by other observations – this physician reasons experimentally, even though he makes no experiments. But if he wishes to go further, and to know the inner mechanism of the disease, he will have to deal with hidden phenomena, and so he will experiment; but he will still reason in the same way.

A naturalist observing animals in all the conditions necessary to their existence, and deducing from these observations consequences verified and controlled by other observations – such a naturalist uses the experimental method even though he performs no experiments, properly speaking. But if he has to go on to observe phenomena inside the stomach, he is forced to invent more or less complex methods of experimentation in order to look inside a cavity hidden from sight. His experimental reasoning, nevertheless, is the same; Réaumur and Spallanzani alike apply the experimental method when making their observations of natural history or their experiments with digestion. When Pascal made a barometric observation at the bottom of the Tour Saint Jacques, and later took another at the top of the tower, we must admit that he performed an experiment; yet here were simply two comparative observations of air pressure carried out in view of the preconceived idea that this pressure should vary according to height. On the other hand, when Jenner, in observing a cuckoo on a tree, used a spy-glass so as not to frighten it, he made a mere observation, because he did not compare this cuckoo with a previous cuckoo, to deduce a conclusion from the observation and to form a judgment about it. In the same way an astronomer first makes observations and then reasons about them to deduce a system of ideas which he controls by observations made in conditions suited to his purpose. The astronomer reasons like an experimenter, because the experience which he gains implies judgment throughout and comparison between two facts bound together in the mind by an idea.

[. . .]

The question remains whether medicine should continue a science of observation or become an experimental science. Medicine must doubtless begin as simple clinical observation. Then, since the human organism is in itself a harmonious unit, a little world (microcosm) contained in the great world (macrocosm), men have actually maintained that life is indivisible and that we should limit ourselves to observing the phenomena presented to us as a whole by living organisms, whether well or sick, and should content ourselves with reasoning on the facts observed. But if we admit that we must so limit ourselves, and if we posit as a principle that medicine is only a passive science of observation, then physicians should no more touch the human body than astronomers touch the planets. Hence, normal and pathological anatomy, vivisection applied to physiology, pathology and therapeutics – all would become completely useless. Medicine so conceived can lead only to prognosis and to hygienic prescriptions of doubtful utility; it is the negation of active medicine, i.e., of real and scientific therapeutics.

[. . .]

Observers and experimenters still have the common and immediate object, in their investigations, of establishing and noting facts and phenomena as rigorously as possible, and with the help of the most appropriate means; they behave exactly as if they were dealing with two ordinary observations. In both cases, indeed, a fact is simply noted; the only difference is this: as the fact which an experimenter must verify does not present itself to him naturally, he must make it appear, i.e. induce it, for a special reason and with a definite object. Hence we may say that an experiment is fundamentally just an observation induced with some object or other. In the experimental method, search for facts, i.e., investigation, is always accompanied by reasoning, so that experimenters usually make an experiment to control or verify the value of an experimental idea. Hence, in this case, the experiment is an observation induced with the object of control.

[. . .]

Men of science who mean to embrace the principles of the experimental method as a whole, must fulfil two classes of conditions and must possess two qualities of mind which are indispensable if they are to reach their goal and succeed in the discovery of truth. First, they must have ideas which they submit to the control of facts; but at the same time they must make sure that the facts which serve as starting point or as control for the idea are correct and well established; they must be at once observers and experimenters.

[. . .]

We said above that the experimental method rests successively on feeling, reason and experiment.

Feeling gives rise to the experimental idea or hypothesis, i.e. the previsioned interpretation of natural phenomena. The whole experimental enterprise comes from the idea, for this it is which induces experiment. Reason or reasoning serves only to deduce the consequences of this idea and to submit them to experiment.

An anticipative idea or an hypothesis is, then, the necessary starting point for all experimental reasoning. Without it, we could not make any investigation at all nor learn anything; we could only pile up sterile observations. If we experimented without a preconceived idea, we should move at random, but, on the other hand, as we have said elsewhere, if we observed with preconceived ideas, we should make bad observations and should risk taking our mental conceptions for reality.

Experimental ideas are by no means innate. They do not arise spontaneously; they must have an outer occasion or stimulant, as is the case in all physiological functions. To have our first idea of things, we must see those things; to have an idea about a natural phenomenon, we must, first of all, observe it. The mind of man cannot conceive an effect without a cause, so that the sight of a phenomenon always awakens an idea of causation. All human knowledge is limited to working back from observed effects to their cause. Following an observation, an idea connected with the cause of the observed phenomenon presents itself to the mind. We then inject this anticipative idea into a train of reasoning, by virtue of which we make experiments to control it.

Experimental ideas, as we shall later see, may arise either *a priori* of a fact observed by chance or following some experimental venture or as corollaries of an accepted theory. For the moment, we may merely note that the experimental idea is by no means arbitrary or purely imaginative; it must always have a support in observed reality, that is to say, in nature. The experimental hypothesis, in short, must always be based on prior observation. Another essential of any hypothesis is that it must be as probable as may be and must be experimentally verifiable. Indeed if we made a hypothesis which experiment could not verify, in that very act we should leave the experimental method to fall into the errors of the scholastics and makers of systems.

Apropos of a given observation, no rules can be given for bringing to birth in the brain a correct and fertile idea that may be a sort of intuitive anticipation of successful research. The idea once set forth, we can only explain how to submit it to the definite precepts and precise rules of logic from which no experimenter may depart; but its appearance is wholly spontaneous, and its nature is wholly individual. A particular feeling, a *quid proprium* constitutes the originality, the inventiveness, or the genius of each man. A new idea appears as a new or unexpected relation which the mind perceives among things. All intellects doubtless resemble each other, and in all men similar ideas may arise in the presence of certain simple relations between things, which everyone can grasp. But like the senses, intellects do not all have the same power or the same acuteness; and subtle and delicate relations exist which can be felt, grasped and unveiled only by minds more perceptive, better endowed or placed in intellectual surroundings which predispose them favorably.

If facts necessarily gave birth to ideas, every new fact ought to beget a new idea. True, this is what most often takes place; for new facts exist, the character of which makes the same new idea come to all men, placed in the same circumstances as respects previous information. But facts also exist which mean nothing to most minds, while they are full of light for others. It even happens that a fact or an observation stays a very long time under the eyes of a man of science without in any way inspiring him; then suddenly there comes a ray of light, and the mind interprets the fact quite differently and finds for it wholly new relations. The new idea appears, then, with the rapidity of lightning, as a kind of sudden revelation, which surely proves that in this case the discovery inheres in a feeling about things which is not only individual, but which is even connected with a transient condition of the mind. The experimental method, then, cannot give new and fruitful ideas to men who have none; it can serve only to guide the ideas of men who have them, to direct their ideas and to develop them so as to get the best possible results. The idea is a seed; the method is the earth furnishing the conditions in which it may develop, flourish and give the best of fruit according to its nature. But as only what has been sown in the ground will ever grow in it, so nothing will be developed by the experimental method except the ideas submitted to it. The method itself gives birth to nothing.

[. . .]

Discovery, then, is a new idea emerging in connection with a fact found by chance or otherwise. Consequently, there can be no method for making discoveries, because philosophic theories can no more give inventive spirit and aptness of mind to men who do not possess them, than knowledge of the laws of acoustics or optics can give a correct ear or good sight to men deprived of them by nature. But good methods can teach us to develop and use to better purpose the faculties with which nature has endowed us, while poor methods may prevent us from turning them to good account. Thus the genius of inventiveness, so precious in the sciences, may be diminished or even smothered by a poor method, while a good method may increase and develop it. In short, a good method promotes scientific development and forewarns men of science against those numberless sources of error which they meet in the search for truth; this is the only possible object of the experimental method. In biological science, the role of method is even more important than in other sciences, because of the immense complexity of the phenomena and the countless sources of error which complexity brings into experimentation.

[. . .]

If a doctor imagined that his reasoning had the value of a mathematician's, he would be utterly in error and would be led into the most unsound conclusions. This is unluckily what has happened and still happens to the men whom I shall call systematizers. These men start, in fact, from an idea which is based more or less on observation, and which they regard as an absolute truth. They then reason logically and without experimenting, and from deduction to deduction they succeed in building a system which is logical, but which has no sort of scientific reality. Superficial persons often let themselves be dazzled by this appearance of logic; and discussions worthy of ancient scholasticism are thus sometimes renewed in our day. The excessive faith in reasoning, which leads physiologists to a false simplification of things, comes, on the one hand, from ignorance of the science of which they speak, and, on the other hand, from lack of a feeling for the complexity of natural phenomena. That is why we sometimes see pure mathematicians, with very great minds too, fall into mistakes of this kind; they simplify too much and reason about phenomena as they construct them in their minds, but not as they exist in nature.

The great experimental principle, then, is doubt – that philosophic doubt which leaves to the mind its freedom and initiative, and from which the virtues most valuable to investigators in physiology and medicine are derived. We must trust our observations or our theories only after experimental verification. If we trust too much, the mind becomes bound and cramped by the results of its own reasoning; it no longer has freedom of action, and so lacks the power to break away from that blind faith in theories which is only scientific superstition.

[. . .]

Men who have excessive faith in their theories or ideas are not only ill-prepared for making discoveries; they also make very poor observations. Of necessity, they observe with a preconceived idea, and when they devise an experiment, they can see, in its results, only a confirmation of their theory. In this way they distort observation and often neglect very important facts because they do not further their aim. This is what made us say elsewhere that we must never make experiments to confirm our ideas, but simply to control them; which means, in other terms, that one must accept the results of experiments as they come, with all their unexpectedness and irregularity.

But it happens further quite naturally that men who believe too firmly in their theories, do not believe enough in the theories of others. So the dominant idea of these despisers of their fellows is to find others' theories faulty and to try to contradict them. The difficulty for science is still the same. They make experiments only to destroy a theory, instead of to seek the truth. At the same time, they make poor observations, because they choose among the results of their experiments only what suits their object, neglecting whatever is unrelated to it, and carefully setting aside everything which might tend toward the idea they wish to combat. By these two opposite roads, men are thus led to the same result, that is, to falsify science and the facts.

Accordingly, we must disregard our own opinion quite as much as the opinion of others, when faced by the decisions of experience. If men discuss and experiment, as we have just said, to prove a preconceived idea in spite of everything, they no longer have freedom of mind, and they no longer search for truth. Theirs is a narrow science, mingled with personal vanity or the diverse passions of man. Pride, however, should have nothing to do with all these vain disputes. When two physiologists or two doctors quarrel, each to maintain his own ideas or theories, in the midst of their contradictory arguments only one thing is absolutely certain: that both theories are insufficient, and neither of them corresponds to the truth. The truly scientific spirit, then, should make us modest and kindly. We really know very little, and we are all fallible when facing the immense difficulties presented by investigation of natural phenomena. The best thing for us to do is to unite our efforts, instead of dividing them and nullifying them by personal disputes. In a word, the man of science wishing to find truth must keep his mind free and calm, and if it be possible, never have his eye bedewed, as Bacon says, by human passions. [. . .]

Physicists and chemists have already often tried to reduce the physico-chemical phenomena of living beings to figures. Among the ancients, as well as among the moderns, the most eminent physicists and chemists wished to establish principles of animal mechanics and laws for chemical statistics of animals. Though the progress of physico-chemical science has made these problems more accessible today than in the past, it seems to me impossible to reach accurate conclusions at present, because foundations are lacking on which to base our calculations. We may, of course, strike a balance between what a living organism takes in as nourishment and what it gives out in excretions; but the results would be mere statistics incapable of throwing light on the inmost phenomena of nutrition in living beings. According to a Dutch chemist's phrase, this would be like trying to tell what happens inside a house by watching what goes in by the door and what comes out by the chimney. [. . .] Let me cite examples of calculations which I condemn, taking them from works which I nevertheless hold in the highest esteem. In 1852 Bidder and Schmidt of Dorpat published highly important works on digestion and nutrition. Their investigations include excellent and very numerous raw data, but in my opinion the deductions from their calculations are often risky or erroneous. Thus, for example, they took a dog weighing 16 kg; in the duct of the submaxillary gland they placed a tube through which the secretion flowed; and in one hour they obtained 5·640 g of saliva, from which they concluded that for both glands this should make 11·280 g. They afterward placed another tube in the duct of the same animal's parotid gland; and in an hour they obtained 8·790 g of saliva which for both parotid glands would make 17·580 g. Now, they went on, if we wish to apply these numbers to man, we must take a man weighing 64 kg or about four times as much as the dog in question; a calculation based on this ratio consequently gives us, for the man's submaxillary glands, 46 g of saliva per hour, or 1·082 kg per day. For the parotid glands, we have 70 g per hour, or 1·687 kg per day which reduced one half gives about 1·40 kg of saliva secreted in twenty-four hours by the salivary glands of an adult man.

As the authors themselves feel, only one thing is true in the above: the crude result found in the dog; all the calculations deduced from this rest on false or doubtful foundations; first of all, doubling the product of one gland to get the product of both is incorrect, because physiology teaches us that in most cases double glands secrete alternately, and that, when one secretes a great deal, the other secretes less; then, besides the two submaxillary and parotid salivary glands, there are others which are not mentioned. Next, it is a mistake to believe that multiplying one hour's output of saliva by twenty-four gives the saliva poured into an animal's mouth in twenty-four hours. In fact, salivary secretion is highly intermittent and takes place only at meal time or when stimulated; during the rest of the time, the secretion is nil or insignificant. Finally, the quantity of saliva got from the salivary glands of the dog in this experiment was not absolute; it would have been nil if the mucous membrane of the mouth had not been stimulated; it might have been greater or less if another stimulant, stronger or weaker than vinegar, had been used.

Now the application of the above calculations to man is still more questionable. If the quantity of saliva had been multiplied by the weight of the salivary glands, a closer relation would have been found; but I cannot concede the validity of calculating the quantity of saliva from the weight of the body taken as a whole. Estimating a phenomenon in kilogrammes of the animal's body seems to me wholly incorrect, when all sorts of tissues foreign to the phenomenon in question are included.

In the part of their investigation devoted to nutrition, Bidder and Schmidt described a very notable experiment, perhaps one of the most laborious ever performed. From the point of view of elementary analysis, they kept a balance sheet of everything taken in and given out by a cat during eight days' nourishment and nineteen days' fasting. But this cat was in a physiological condition of which they were unaware; she was pregnant, and she had her kittens on the seventeenth day of the experiment. In these circumstances, our authors considered the kittens as excretions, and calculated them with other eliminated materials as a simple loss of weight. I believe that these interpretations should be rectified when trying to define such complex phenomena.

[. . .]

Chemico-physical phenomena of living organisms are therefore still too complex today to be embraced as a whole, except by means of hypotheses. To find correct solutions of such vast problems, we must begin by analysing the results of complicated reactions, and by separating them experimentally into distinct and simple questions. In several attempts which I have made on this analytic path, I have shown that we should not handle the problem of nutrition *en bloc*, but rather should first define the nature of the physico-chemical phenomena taking place in an organ made of some definite tissue, such as a muscle, gland or nerve; that we must at the same time take account of the organ's state of activity or rest. I have also shown that we can regulate an organ's state of rest or activity at will, by means of its nerves, and that we can even act on it locally without reverberation through the organism, if we first separate the peripheral nerves from the nervous centres. When we have analysed the physico-chemical phenomena peculiar to each tissue and each organ, then only can we try to understand nutrition as a whole and to found biochemistry on a solid base, that is to say, on the study of definite, complete and comparable physiological facts.

[. . .]

Chemical averages are also often used. If we collect a man's urine during twenty-four hours and mix all this urine to analyse the average, we get an analysis of a urine which simply does not exist; for urine, when fasting, is different from urine during digestion. A startling instance of this kind was invented by a physiologist who took urine from a railroad station urinal where people of all nations passed, and who believed he could thus present an analysis of *average* European urine!

Robert Koch

Although bacteria had been observed in the seventeenth century, soon after the invention of the microscope, the relation between bacteria and disease was not demonstrated until relatively late in the nineteenth century. Robert Koch (1842–1910) devoted himself to studying this relationship, and in his work he proved the specific bacterial cause for several important diseases, devised techniques of incalculable value, defined methodological principles, and trained productive investigators who brought further illumination to medical science.

Koch, after an excellent preliminary education, graduated MD from Göttingen in 1866, and then, following further clinical training in army service in the Franco-Prussian war, settled in East Prussia as a country practitioner and 'district surgeon'. He had a successful clinical practice but he also set up his own private laboratory where, in his spare time, he carried out his researches.

His first great contribution was his study on anthrax. Using mice as the experimental animal, he transmitted the disease serially, demonstrated spore formation in the bacteria and properly interpreted its role, made pure cultures of the organism outside the living body (the first time this had ever been done for a pathogenic organism) and established the bacterium as the specific cause of the disease. Even with his primitive techniques his work was so skilful that to this day it forms the basis of our knowledge of anthrax.

His studies, published in 1876, attracted immediate attention and at once marked him as a brilliant investigator. When he wrote, only one other disease – relapsing fever – had been definitely traced to a specific bacterium. We can thus appreciate the giant step that Koch had taken when he established the pathogenesis of anthrax. Other steps followed quickly. In 1878 he published an important study on the infections that resulted from wounds. He showed experimentally that putrid substances, injected into animals, produced a whole series of diseases, correlated with particular micro-organisms; furthermore, he distinguished pathogenic from non-pathogenic bacteria. In other works he described many technical innovations in bacteriology, including staining techniques and culture methods, particularly those for isolating pure cultures.

His epoch-making work on the tubercle bacillus and its relation to the disease tuberculosis appeared in 1882. Tuberculosis can take many different forms, so varied that they may appear clinically as quite distinct diseases – e.g. 'consumption', scrofula, and Pott's disease. Were these, and numerous other forms, manifestations of the same disease? How could you prove it? If bacteria were discovered, were they truly causal or merely casual? And how could you tell? Koch's studies, directed toward these questions, depended on new technical methods that he devised, which permitted him to demonstrate the bacillus both in stained preparations and in pure culture. His conceptual analysis, known since as Koch's postulates, set up criteria for asserting a causal relationship between microbial agents and disease.

In the next two years Koch and his associates demonstrated the bacterial causes for glanders, Asiatic cholera, diphtheria and typhoid. Other workers added further diseases to a growing list. Indeed, the years 1881 to 1900 represented the 'etiological period' of bacteriology, a sort of golden age when specific agents for many infectious diseases were being discovered, and high hopes were raised for the conquest of all disease.

Koch's life was by no means a succession of uninterrupted triumphs. His studies on tuberculin led to particular disappointment, but his errors are insignificant compared with his achievements. He received the Nobel Prize for Medicine in 1905.

The 1882 study on tuberculosis, from which the present excerpts are taken, has particular importance. Koch devised a new staining method and new culture methods that could identify the tubercle bacillus, and he showed that tuberculosis was a 'parasitic disease' resulting from infections with this specific bacterium. And this bacillus he proved to be the inciting etiologic agent. By identifying this agent he gave a precise definition to the disease and demonstrated the similarity of all the different manifestations. His experimental work and his conceptual analysis exemplified medical science at its best.

21 The Etiology of Tuberculosis (1882)

Excerpts from R. Koch, 'The Etiology of Tuberculosis', in *Medical Classics*, vol. 2, 1938, no. 8, pp. 853–79.

[. . .]

If the number of victims which a disease claims is taken as a measure of its importance, then all diseases, especially the most feared contagious diseases, plague, cholera, etc., must take a place far behind that of tuberculosis. Statistics show that one seventh of all people die of tuberculosis, and if only the productive middle aged class is considered, tuberculosis carries away a third and often more of these.

[. . .]

Attempts have been made repeatedly to investigate the nature of tuberculosis thoroughly, but up to now they have been fruitless. The so frequently successful staining methods used for the demonstration of pathogenic micro-organisms have left this disease in the lurch, and the attempts made to isolate and cultivate the virus of tuberculosis up to the present can not be regarded as successful.

[. . .]

The aim of the investigations had to be directed first toward the demonstration of some sort of parasitic organism foreign to the body, which possibly could be explained as the cause of the disease. This demonstration was indeed carried out successfully by means of a certain staining method, with the aid of which characteristic bacteria, previously unknown, were found in all organs affected by tuberculosis. [There follows a technical description of the staining process.]

The bacteria made visible by this method show a behaviour which, in many respects, is characteristic. They have a rod-shaped form and thus belong to the group of bacilli. They are very thin and are from a quarter to one-half of the diameter of a red blood corpuscle in length; however, at times they attain greater length, up to the full diameter of a red blood cell. [. . .] The bacilli are present in large numbers in all situations where the tuberculous process is early in origin and making rapid progress; they then usually form little groups which are pressed closely together and at times are arranged in bundles. Many times these lie within cells and present a picture like that of lepra bacilli heaped within the cells. On the other hand, many free bacilli are found. Particularly on the borders of large caseous foci, crowds of bacilli which are not inclosed in cells are found.

As soon as the height of the tuberculous process is passed the bacilli become more rare, are found only in small groups or entirely alone on the edges of tuberculous foci, [. . .]. Finally, they may disappear completely, yet they are rarely entirely absent and then only in those cases in which the tuberculous process is arrested. If giant cells are present in the tuberculous tissue, then the bacilli lie chiefly within these structures.

[. . .]

Under certain conditions, to be mentioned later, the bacilli form spores, even in the animal body; and indeed, the single bacillus contains several, usually two to four spores of oval form which are distributed throughout its length.

In regard to the presence of the bacilli in the various tuberculous processes in man and animals the following material has been observed.

1. *Human.* Eleven cases of miliary tuberculosis. The bacilli were never lacking in the miliary tubercles in the lungs; [. . .]. Beside the lungs they could be demonstrated in miliary tubercles of the spleen, liver and kidneys. They were present in abundance in the gray nodules of the pia mater in basilar meningitis. Also, in several cases examined, the caseous bronchial glands contained, in part, dense swarms of bacilli [. . .].

Twelve cases of caseous bronchitis and pneumonia (cavity formation in six cases). The presence of the bacilli was limited chiefly to the edges of the caseous, infiltrated tissues, but they were frequently very abundant. [. . .]

One case of solitary tubercle of the brain, larger than a hazel nut. The caseous mass of the tubercle was surrounded by cellular tissue in which many giant cells were embedded. The majority of giant cells contained no parasites, but occasionally groups of giant cell each containing one or two bacilli were met.

Two cases of intestinal tuberculosis. In the tubercles grouped about the intestinal ulcers, the bacilli could be demonstrated especially well, and indeed, here again they were found particularly numerous in the most recent and smallest nodules.

Three cases of recently excised scrofulous lymph nodes. In only two of these could bacilli inclosed in giant cells be demonstrated.

Four cases of proliferative arthritis. In two cases bacilli were found but only in small isolated groups of giant cells.

2. *In animals.* Ten cases of bovine tuberculosis with calcified nodules in the lungs, several also in the peritoneum, and, in one case, on the pericardium. In all cases the bacilli were present, principally within the giant cells which were in the tissue surrounding the calcified masses. [. . .]

Three cases in which the lungs of cattle did not contain the usual calcified nodules with uneven surfaces of the usual tuberculosis, but on the contrary, smooth walled, round nodules filled with thick, soupy, cheesy material. Usually this form is not regarded as tuberculosis, but as bronchiectasis. However, in the vicinity of these nodules, giant cells were found and in them the tubercle bacilli.

One caseous cervical lymph node of a pig contained the bacilli.

In the organs of a fowl dead of tuberculosis, and, indeed, in tubercles of the bone marrow, as well as in the peculiar nodules of the intestines, liver and lungs, large numbers of bacilli were found.

In three monkeys, spontaneously dead of tuberculosis, the lungs, spleen, liver, omentum, which were riddled with countless nodules, and the caseous lymph nodes, were examined and tubercle bacilli found in all the nodules or in their immediate vicinity.

Of spontaneously ill animals, nine guinea-pigs and seven rabbits came to examination, which disclosed the bacilli everywhere in the tubercles.

Beside these cases of spontaneous tuberculosis, there was provided for me a not inconsiderable number of animals which were infected by means of inoculation with various tuberculous substances; [. . .]. The number of animals infected in this way amounts to 172 guinea-pigs, 32 rabbits and 5 cats. The demonstration of the bacilli in the majority of these cases had to be limited to examination of the tubercles of the lungs which were always present in large numbers. In these the bacilli were not absent a single time; [. . .].

It is striking that in spite of the regularity of the occurrence of the tubercle bacilli, no one up to the present has seen them. Yet this can be explained by the fact that the bacilli are extraordinarily tiny structures and for the most part are so scant in number, especially when their presence is limited to the interior of the giant cells, that without special staining methods they must escape the most careful observer. Even though they are present in large numbers, they are mixed with finely granular detritis and obscured by it in such a way that their recognition is extremely difficult.

Moreover, there are several accounts of micro-organisms having been found in tissues showing the changes of tuberculosis. Thus Schüller mentions in his paper on scrofulous and tuberculous joint diseases that he has found micrococci constantly. Doubtless we are concerned here, just as in the case of Klebs, who found extremely tiny motile granules in tubercles, with something other than the tubercle bacilli which I observed, and which are non-motile and rod shaped. [He gives other examples.]

On the basis of my numerous observations I state it to be proved that the bacteria designated by me as the tubercle bacilli are present in all cases of tuberculous disease of man and animals, and that they may be differentiated from all other micro-organisms by their characteristic properties. It does not necessarily follow from this coincidence of the tuberculous disease and the bacilli that the two phenomena have an original association, although no small amount of probability is given to this theory by the fact the bacilli are found chiefly where the process is beginning or progressing, and that they disappear in those places where the disease comes to a standstill.

In order to prove that tuberculosis is a parasitic disease caused by the invasion of the bacilli and primarily influenced by the growth and proliferation of the latter, the bacilli had to be isolated from the body and cultivated in pure culture until devoid of all adherent products of disease originating from the animal organism; and, finally, through transfer of the isolated bacilli to animals, the same clinical picture of tuberculosis as is obtained empirically by the injection of naturally developed tuberculous material had to be produced.

[He describes the technique of culture.]

The cultures resulting from the growth of tubercle bacilli first appear to the naked eye in the second week after inoculation, usually not until after the tenth day, as very tiny points and dry scales. [. . .] If only a very few bacilli were present in the material inoculated, then it is hardly ever possible to free the bacilli from the tissue and bring them into direct contact with the culture medium. In this case they develop their colonies within the bits of tissue and if this is transparent enough – if, for example, it is in small pieces which have been taken from scrofulous glands – whitish, shining points may be seen within it when the light strikes it. [. . .] The markedly slow growth which is attained only at incubator temperature, the peculiarly dry and scale like condition of these bacillary colonies occur in no other known type of bacteria, so that confusion of the cultures of tubercle bacilli with those of other bacteria is impossible; and after only a small amount of practice nothing is easier to detect at once than accidental contamination of the cultures.

[. . .]

Among hundreds of recently bought guinea-pigs, which opportunely came to autopsy in the course of other experiments, I have never found a single tuberculous one. Spontaneous tuberculosis always occurred in isolated instances and never before the course of three to four months during which time the animals had been in the same room with those infected with tuberculosis. In animals spontaneously ill of tuberculosis, I found the bronchial lymph nodes, without exception, to be uncommonly large and broken down into pus and usually in the lungs also a large caseous focus with far advanced necrosis in the centre, so that several times true cavity formation had taken place exactly as in human lungs. The development of tubercles in the abdominal viscera lagged far behind that in the lungs. [. . .] Inoculation tuberculosis acts in an entirely different manner. The site of inoculation in these animals was in the belly in the vicinity of the inguinal lymph nodes. These swelled first of all and thereby gave an early and infallible sign as to the success of the inoculation. The tuberculosis ran a much more rapid course than the spontaneous tuberculosis, because to begin with, a larger amount of infectious material was taken into the body; and on section of these animals, the spleen and liver showed far more changes of tuberculosis than did the lungs. Thus it is not at all difficult to differentiate spontaneous tuberculosis from inoculation tuberculosis in laboratory animals.

[. . .]

The results were uniform throughout. In all animals which were inoculated with fresh material containing tubercle bacilli the tiny injection wound was almost always crusted over on the following day. It remained unchanged for about eight days, then a nodule formed which either enlarged without breaking down or, as was the usual case, developed into a flat dry ulcer. Within two weeks the inguinal nodes on the side of the inoculation wound, at times also the axillary nodes, were enlarged to pea size. From then on the animals quickly became emaciated, and died after four to six weeks, or were killed in order to avoid any combination with a later developing spontaneous tuberculosis. In the organs of all these animals, and chiefly in the spleen and liver, the characteristic, well-known tuberculous changes of guinea-pigs were found. That, indeed, the infection of the guinea-pigs in this series of experiments resulted only from the injected material is demonstrated by the fact that, in other series of experiments with inoculation of a scrofulous gland, and fungous material from a joint in which no tubercle bacilli could be found, and after injections of pulmonary tubercles (monkey), which had been dried for two months and with some which had been kept in alcohol for a month, not a single one of the animals inoculated became ill, while those injected with material containing bacilli showed marked tuberculosis in four weeks without exception.

From such guinea-pigs as had been infected by inoculation with tubercles from the lungs of monkeys, with miliary tubercles from the brain and lungs of humans, with caseous material from phthisical lungs and with nodes from the lungs and peritoneum of tuberculous cattle, cultures of tubercle bacilli were obtained in the manner previously described. As a result, it was found that, just as the clinical picture which the various substances enumerated produced in the guinea-pigs never varied, so the cultures of bacilli obtained did not differ from one another in the slightest degree. In all, fifteen such pure cultures of tubercle bacilli were obtained and of these four were from guinea-pigs which were infected with tuberculosis from monkeys, four with bovine tuberculosis and seven with tuberculous material from humans.

However, in order to exclude any possible objection that a change in the nature of the bacilli, possibly a bringing about of similarity between previously dissimilar organisms, was caused by the inoculation of the tuberculous material into the guinea-pigs, an attempt was made to cultivate the tubercle bacilli directly from the spontaneously diseased organs of humans and animals.

This experiment succeeded many times and pure cultures were obtained from two human lungs with miliary tuberculosis, from another with caseous pneumonia, twice from the contents of small cavities of phthisical lungs, once from caseous mesenteric nodes and twice from freshly extirpated scrofulous nodes, in addition, twice from the lungs of cattle with bovine tuberculosis and three times from the lungs of guinea-pigs spontaneously ill of tuberculosis. Moreover, these cultures were entirely similar to one another, just as were those obtained by the roundabout method of inoculating guinea-pigs, so that the unity of identity of the bacilli present in the various tuberculous processes can not be doubted.

[. . .]

Thus, up to this point, my investigations have established that the presence of characteristic bacilli is regularly bound up with tuberculosis and that these bacilli can be obtained from tuberculous organs and isolated in pure culture. It now remained to answer the weighty question as to whether the isolated bacilli if again introduced into the body, are able to produce the pathological processes of tuberculosis.

In order to exclude any error from the solution of this question, wherein lies the crux of the whole investigation of the tubercle virus, series of experiments, as varied as possible, were set up and shall be enumerated in detail because of the significance of the point in question.

First, experiments with simple inoculation of the bacilli in the manner previously described were set up.

Experiment 1 Of six newly bought guinea-pigs which were kept in the same cage, four were inoculated on the abdomen with cultures of bacilli obtained from human lungs with miliary tuberculosis and cultivated for 54 days through five changes of culture material. Two animals remained uninjected. After 14 days the inguinal nodes of the inoculated animals swelled, the sites of injection ulcerated and the animals became emaciated. After 32 days one of the animals inoculated died. After 35 days the remainder of the animals were killed. The injected animals, the one which had died as well as the three which were killed, showed advanced tuberculosis of the spleen, liver and lungs; the inguinal nodes were greatly swollen and caseous, the bronchial nodes but slightly swollen. Neither of the animals which were not injected showed the slightest trace of tuberculosis in the lungs, the liver or the spleen.

Experiment 2 Of eight guinea-pigs, six were inoculated with cultures of bacilli which originated from the tuberculous lungs of monkeys and were cultivated for 95 days with eight transfers. Two animals remained uninjected for controls. The course was exactly the same as in the first experiment. The six injected animals showed advanced tuberculosis at autopsy; the two uninjected ones were found healthy when they were killed after 32 days.

Experiment 3 Of six guinea-pigs, five were inoculated with cultures arising from a lung of bovine tuberculosis, 72 days old, transferred six times. The five injected animals were found tuberculous, the uninjected ones healthy, after 34 days when all the animals were killed.

Experiment 4 A number of animals (mice, rats, hedgehogs, a hamster, pigeons, frogs) whose susceptibility to tuberculosis is not known, were inoculated with cultures obtained from the tuberculous lung of a monkey and cultivated for 113 days outside of the animal body. Four field mice, killed 53 days after injection, had numerous tubercles in the spleen, liver and lungs, as did the hamster, killed 53 days after inoculation.

In these first four experiments the inoculation of cultures of bacilli on the abdomen of the experimental animals has thus produced the same clinical picture of tuberculosis as when fresh tuberculous material had been injected.

[Other experiments are recounted in comparable detail.]

If one looks back over these experiments, it is apparent that a not inconsiderable number of experimental animals that had received the cultures of bacilli in various ways, that is, by simple inoculation into the subcutaneous tissue, through injection into the abdominal cavity, or into the anterior chamber of the eye or directly into the blood stream, had been rendered tuberculous without a single exception; and, indeed, had not developed only a solitary tubercle but the extraordinary number of tubercles was proportionate to the large number of infectious germs introduced. In other animals it was possible by the injection of a minimal number of bacilli into the anterior chamber of the eye, to produce a tuberculous iritis, [. . .].

A confusion with spontaneous tuberculosis or an accidental unintentional infection of the experimental animals in these experiments is excluded on the following grounds. First of all, neither spontaneous tuberculosis nor an accidental infection can cause this massive eruption of tubercles in so short a space of time. Secondly, the control animals which were treated in exactly the same manner as the infected animals, with the single difference, that they received no culture of bacilli, remained healthy. Thirdly, this typical picture of miliary tuberculosis never occurred in numerous guinea-pigs and rabbits injected and infected in the same way with other substances for other experimental purposes, as it then only arises when the body is overcome to a certain extent by a large amount of infectious germs at one time.

All these facts, taken together, substantiate the claim that the bacilli present in tuberculous material, not only accompany the tuberculous process, but are actually the cause of it, and that, in these bacilli, we have the true virus of tuberculosis.

Thus it is also made possible to delimit what diseases shall be understood as tuberculosis, which up to now could not be done with certainty. A definite criterion for tuberculosis was lacking and one person included miliary tuberculosis, phthisis, scrofula, bovine tuberculosis, etc., while another, perhaps just as correctly, regarded all these processes as different. In the future it will not be difficult to decide what is tuberculous and what is not. Not the peculiar structure of the tubercles, not the presence of giant cells, will settle the question, but the demonstration of tubercle bacilli, whether it be in the tissues by the staining reactions or whether it be by culture on solidified blood serum. Accepting this criterion as standard, miliary tuberculosis, caseous pneumonia, caseous bronchitis, intestinal and glandular tuberculosis, bovine tuberculosis and spontaneous and inoculation tuberculosis in animals must be declared identical as the result of my investigations. [. . .]

Having established the parasitic nature of tuberculosis, it must be determined from whence the parasites come and how they gain entrance to the body, in order to answer completely the question as to etiology.

In regard to the first question, it is necessary to discover whether the infectious material will develop only under the conditions existing in the animal body, or whether it can develop in any stage free in nature, as, for example, the anthrax bacillus is independent of the animal organism.

It was now determined by many experiments that the tubercle bacilli grow only in temperatures between 30 and 41°C. Below 30°C, just as at 42°C, the slightest growth did not occur within three weeks, while anthrax bacilli, for example, grow vigorously even at 20°C and between 42 and 43°C. On the basis of this one fact, the questions raised can be decided. In the temperate climate, with the exception of the animal body, no opportunity is offered for a uniform temperature of over 30°C of at least two weeks duration. From this it follows, that the tubercle bacilli must turn to the animal organism exclusively in their developmental processes; thus, they are not occasional parasites but true parasites and can arise only from the animal organism.

The second question as to how the parasites enter the body is also answered. The vast majority of all cases of tuberculosis have their origin in the respiratory passages and the infectious material first makes itself manifest in the lungs or in the bronchial nodes. Thus it is also highly probable that the tubercle bacilli are usually inhaled with the inspired air, clinging to particles of dust. There can be no doubt as to the manner in which they reach the air if one considers in what large quantities the tubercle bacilli, present in the contents of cavities of patients with pulmonary tuberculosis, must be expectorated with the sputum and thus spread all about.

[. . .]

If we now ask what further significance the results obtained in this investigation of tuberculosis have, then it is to be regarded as a victory for science that it has been successful, for the first time, in furnishing complete proof of the parasitic nature of a human infectious disease; indeed, of the most important one of all. Up to now such proof had been established only for anthrax, while for a number of infectious diseases affecting man – for example, relapsing fever, wound infection, leprosy, gonorrhea – the simultaneous presence of the parasite with the pathologic process was known without being able to prove the causal relationship between the two. It can be expected that the explanation of the etiology of tuberculosis will produce new points of view for the forming of opinions regarding the other infectious diseases, and that the methods of investigation, which have been used successfully in seeking out the etiology of tuberculosis, will be of use in working out the other infectious diseases.

Walter Reed

To conquer an infectious disease, we must first of all know a great deal about it. Does it have a unique inciting agent? A definite and specific mode of spread? A predictable symptomatology and course? Special predisposing or contributory factors? If we can find specific answers to these questions, then we may be able to break the chain of causation and control the disease. But to achieve success the answers must be scrupulously accurate. Medical science must provide the necessary degree of accuracy.

Yellow fever was a great scourge. But although it had been extensively studied, none of the important questions had received satisfactory answers. Walter Reed and his co-workers, in a series of superb experiments, found rigorous answers that have enabled us to control the disease.

Considerable evidence, already on record, had pointed to the mosquito as having a role in transmitting the naturally occuring disease. But the attendant circumstances were not clearly understood. Was the mosquito the only mode of natural transmission or could the disease spread by other means as well, e.g., through direct contact or through fomites and dejecta? Reed and his fellow investigators had to work out an experimental design that would give definite and unequivocal answers.

To achieve their goals the researchers had to plan their experiments, anticipate possible objections, and find means of eliminating the objections. This required precise controls for every important step. To study the transmission of disease, the investigators had to have susceptible subjects, and only human volunteers could serve. Since an attack of yellow fever conferred an immunity, Reed needed subjects who had never had the disease; and as controls, he needed those who were already immune. We must realize that there were at that time no sharp criteria whereby physicians could diagnose yellow fever. Today we are accustomed to highly specific tests that can, in many conditions, accurately identify the presence of a particular disease, through demonstration of the agent itself or antibodies thereto.

But Reed had no such criteria for yellow fever. Diagnosis depended on clinical judgment. The patient was considered to have yellow fever when a skilled and experienced clinician said that he did.

To evaluate the role of the mosquito, Reed had to have situations where the insect was the only link between a known case of the disease and a susceptible subject; and he also had to perform the reverse experiment, where there were many links such as indirect contacts, but where mosquitos were rigidly excluded. In the first instance, he had to show that the volunteers bitten by the mosquitos contracted the disease, while immune patients did not. In the second instance, he had to show that the volunteers did not contract yellow fever from contact with fomites and dejecta of yellow-fever patients, and he also had to show that the same volunteers would contract the disease if subsequently bitten by an infectious mosquito. And furthermore, he had to define the interval required for a mosquito to become infectious after it had bitten a yellow-fever patient.

The brilliant way in which Reed and his colleagues proved their points, and set up adequate controls to eliminate other possibilities, forms a masterpiece in the literature of science.

22 The Etiology of Yellow Fever (1901)

Excerpts from W. Reed, J. Carroll and A. Agramonte, 'The Etiology of Yellow Fever, An Additional Note', *Journal of the American Medical Association*, 16 February 1901, pp. 431–40.

At the Twenty-eighth Annual Meeting of the American Public Health Association, held in Indianapolis, Ind., 22–6 October 1900, we presented, in the form of a preliminary note, the results of our bacteriologic study of yellow fever, based on cultures taken from the blood in eighteen cases, at various stages of the disease, as well as on those which we had made from the blood and organs of eleven yellow fever cadavers. We also recorded the results obtained from the inoculation of eleven non-immune individuals by means of the bite of mosquitoes (*Culex fasciatus, Fabr.*) that had previously fed on the blood of patients sick with yellow fever. We were able to report two positive results, in which the attack of yellow fever followed the bite of a mosquito within the usual period of incubation of this disease.

In one of these cases all other sources of infection could be positively excluded. From our several observations we drew the following conclusions: 1. Bacillus icteroides (Sanarelli) stands in no causative relation to yellow fever, but, when present, should be considered as a secondary invader in this disease. 2. The mosquito serves as the intermediate host for the parasite of yellow fever. Since the publication of our preliminary note, we have continued our investigations, especially as regards the means by which yellow fever is propagated from individual to individual, and as to the manner in which houses become infected with the contagium of this disease. [. . .]

In order to exercise perfect control over the movements of those individuals who were to be subjected to experimentation, and to avoid any other possible source of infection, a location was selected in an open and uncultivated field, about one mile from the town of Quemados, Cuba. Here an experimental sanitary station was established under the complete control of the senior member of this Board. This station was named Camp Lazear, in honor of our late colleague, Dr Jesse W. Lazear, Acting Assistant-Surgeon, USA, who died of yellow fever while courageously investigating the causation of this disease. The site selected was very well drained, freely exposed to sunlight and winds, and, from every point of view, satisfactory for the purposes intended.

The personnel of this camp consisted of two medical officers, Dr Roger P. Ames, Acting Assistant-Surgeon, USA, an immune, in immediate charge; Dr R. P. Cooke, Acting Assistant-Surgeon, USA, non-immune; one acting hospital steward, an immune; nine privates of the hospital corps, one of whom was immune, and one immune ambulance driver.

For the quartering of this detachment, and of such non-immune individuals as should be received for experimentation, hospital tents, properly floored, were provided. These were placed at a distance of about twenty feet from each other, and were numbered 1 to 7 respectively.

Camp Lazear was established on 20 November 1900, and from this date was strictly quarantined, no one being permitted to leave or enter camp except the three immune members of the detachment and the members of the Board. Supplies were drawn chiefly from Columbia Barracks, and for this purpose a conveyance under the control of an immune acting hospital steward, and having an immune driver, was used.

A few Spanish immigrants recently arrived at the Port of Havana, were received at Camp Lazear, from time to time, while these observations were being carried out. A non-immune person, having once left this camp, was not permitted to return to it under any circumstances whatever.

The temperature and pulse of all non-immune residents were carefully recorded three times a day. Under these circumstances any infected individual entering the camp could be promptly detected and removed. As a matter of fact only two persons, not the subject of experimentation, developed any rise of temperature; one, a Spanish immigrant, with probably commencing pulmonary tuberculosis, who was discharged at the end of three days; and the other, a Spanish immigrant, who developed a temperature of 102·6°F on the afternoon of his fourth day in camp. He was at once removed with his entire bedding and baggage and placed in the receiving ward at Columbia Barracks. His fever, which was marked by daily intermissions for three days, subsided upon the administration of cathartics and enemata. His attack was considered to be due to intestinal irritation. He was not permitted, however, to return to the camp.

No non-immune resident was subjected to inoculation who had not passed in this camp the full period of incubation of yellow fever, with one exception, to be hereinafter mentioned.

Observations

[. . .] At the time these inoculations were begun, the several tents were occupied as follows: tent no. 1 by one immune and one non-immune; no. 2 by one immune and two non-immunes; no. 3 by two immunes; no. 4 by three non-immunes; no. 5 by three non-immunes; no. 6 by two non-immunes; and no. 7 by one non-immune.

For the purpose of experimentation subjects were selected as follows: from tent no. 2, two non-immunes, and from tent no. 5, three non-immunes. Later, one non-immune in tent no. 6 was also designated for inoculation.

Case 1. Private John R. Kissinger, Hospital Corps, USA, aged 23, a non-immune, occupant of tent no. 2, with his full consent, was bitten at 10.30 a.m., 20 November 1900, by a mosquito – *C. fasciatus* – that had bitten a severe case of yellow fever on the fifth day, eleven days previously; another severe case, on the third day, six days before, and a third severe one on the third day, three days before. As Kissinger had not absented himself from Columbia Barracks for a period of more than thirty days, it was considered safe to inoculate him without waiting for his period of incubation to pass.

23 November 1900, Kissinger was again bitten by the same mosquito. The result of both inoculations was negative. The mosquito, therefore, was incapable of conveying any infection on the eleventh or fourteenth day after it had bitten a severe case of yellow fever on the third day of the disease. This insect had been kept at ordinary room temperature and died 26 November 1900.

5 December 1900, at 2 p.m., twelve days after the last inoculation, Kissinger was again bitten by five mosquitoes – *C. fasciatus* – two of which had bitten fatal cases of yellow fever, on the second day, fifteen days before; one a severe case on the second day, nineteen days previously, and two a mild case on the third day, twenty-one days before.

The record of temperature and pulse, taken every three hours, following this inoculation, showed that the subject remained in his usual state of health during the following three days, except that on 8 December, on the third day, Kissinger had slight vertigo, upon rising, which soon passed away. At 4.30 p.m. – commencement of fourth day – he complained of frontal headache; otherwise he felt well and partook of supper with appetite; at 9 p.m., temperature was 98·4°F, pulse 90; at 11.30 p.m., he awoke with a chill, his temperature 100°F, pulse 90; he complained of severe frontal headache and backache; his eyes were injected and his face suffused. 9 December at 3 a.m., his temperature was 102°F, pulse 102; he had violent headache and backache with nausea and vomiting. He was then removed to the yellow fever wards. His subsequent history was that of a case of yellow fever at moderate severity. The diagnosis of yellow fever in this case was made by Drs Juan Guitéras, Carlos Finlay, W. C. Gorgas, and A. Diaz Albertini, the board of yellow fever experts of the city of Havana, who saw the patient on several occasions during his illness. The period of incubation in this case was 3 days, 9½ hours.

Case 2. John J. Moran, aged 24, an American, non-immune occupant of tent no. 2, with his full consent, was bitten at 10 a.m., 26 November 1900, by a mosquito – *C. fasciatus* – which twelve days before had bitten a case of yellow fever of moderate severity, on the third day of the disease This insect had also bitten a well-marked case of yellow fever – second day – ten days previously.

29 November, at 2.20 p.m., Moran was again bitten by the same mosquito. The result of both these inoculations was negative. This insect, was, therefore, incapable of conveying the infection fifteen days after having bitten a case of yellow fever of moderate severity on the third day, and thirteen days after it had bitten a well-marked case of this disease on the second day. This mosquito had been kept at room temperature. Moran's case will be again referred to when we come to speak of the infection of a building by means of contaminated mosquitoes.

Case 3. A Spanish immigrant, aged 26, a non-immune occupant of tent no. 5, with his full consent, was bitten at 4 p.m., 8 December 1900, by four mosquitoes – *C. fasciatus* – which had been contaminated as follows: one by biting a fatal case of yellow fever, on the third day, seventeen days before; one a severe one, on the third day, eighteen days before; one a severe case, on the second day, twenty-two days before, and one a case of moderate severity, on the third day, twenty-four days previously.

The record of temperature and pulse, taken every three hours after the inoculation, shows no rise of temperature above 99°F until 6 p.m., 13 December, on the sixth day, when 99·4°F is recorded; pulse 68. The subject, who was of a very lively disposition, retained his usual spirits until noon of the 13th, although he complained of slight frontal headache on the 11th and 12th. He took to his bed at noon of the 13th, the fifth day, complaining of increased frontal headache and a sense of fatigue. At 9 p.m., his temperature was 98·2°F, pulse 62.

14 December, at 6 a.m., temperature was 98°F, pulse 72, and he still complained of frontal headache and general malaise. Profuse epistaxis occurred at 7.45 a.m.; at 9 a.m., temperature was 99·6°F, pulse 80; at 1.15 p.m., temperature was 100°F, pulse 80, and he complained of a sense of chilliness, with frontal headache increased, and slight pain in the back, arms and legs; at 3 p.m., temperature was 100°F, pulse 80; at 4.15 p.m., temperature 100·7°F, pulse 68; his face flushed and eyes congested. He was removed to the yellow fever wards. A trace of albumin was found in the urine passed at 3.30 p.m., 15 December; a few hyaline cases were present. He was seen at this time by the Havana board of experts and the diagnosis of mild yellow fever confirmed.

The period of incubation in this case was four days and twenty hours, counting from the time of inoculation to the hour when the patient took to his bed; if reckoned to the onset of fever, it was 5 days, 17 hours.

Case 4. A Spanish immigrant, aged 27, a non-immune occupant of tent no. 5, with his full consent, was bitten at 10 a.m., 26 November 1900, by a mosquito – *C. fasciatus* – which had bitten a severe case of yellow fever, on the second day, ten days before. Three days later, 29 November, he was again bitten by the same insect. 2 December, after an interval of three days, he was again bitten by the same insect, and also by a second mosquito – *C. fasciatus* – which, twelve days before, had been contaminated by biting a fatal case of yellow fever on the third day. No unfavorable effects followed any of these attempted inoculations. The first-mentioned mosquito, therefore, was incapable of conveying any infection on the seventeenth day after biting a severe case of yellow fever on the second day; the other also failed to infect on the twelfth day after biting a fatal case of yellow fever on the third day. Both of these mosquitoes had been kept at ordinary room temperature.

9 December, after an interval of seven days, the subject was again bitten, at 10.30 a.m., by one mosquito – *C. fasciatus* – which had been infected nineteen days before by biting a fatal case of yellow fever on the second day of the disease. He remained in his usual health until 9 a.m., 12 December, the third day, when he complained of frontal headache; his temperature was 98·8°F, pulse 96. This headache continued during the entire day. At 6 p.m., temperature was 99°F, pulse 94; at 9 p.m., temperature 99°F, pulse 84; at 9.30 p.m., temperature 99·4°F, pulse 82. Severe headache and backache was complained of; his eyes

were injected and his face suffused. The following morning he was sent to the yellow-fever wards. [. . .]

The patient was seen by the board of experts on 14 December, and the diagnosis of yellow fever made.

The period of incubation in this case was 3 days, $11\frac{1}{2}$ hours.

Case 5. A Spanish immigrant, aged 26, a non-immune occupant of tent no. 5, with his full consent, was bitten at 10 a.m., 26 November 1900, by a mosquito – *C. fasciatus* – that had bitten a well-marked case of yellow fever, on the third day, twelve days before. 29 November he was again bitten by the same insect. 2 December he was for the third time bitten by two mosquitoes – *C. fasciatus* – both of which had bitten a well-marked case of yellow fever, on the third day, eighteen days before. As no bad results followed any of these inoculations, it follows that these mosquitoes were incapable of conveying any infection eighteen days after they had bitten a well-marked case of yellow fever on the third day. Both of these insects had been kept at room temperature.

11 December, after an interval of nine days, the subject was again, at 4.30 p.m., bitten by the same mosquitoes, four in number, that had been applied to Case 3, three days prior to this time, with positive results.

The record of temperature and pulse, taken every three hours following the inoculation, showed no change till 13 December, the second day, at 9 a.m., when the temperature was 99°F, and the pulse 78. From this hour till 6 p.m. the temperature varied from 99·2 to 99·6°F. The subject complained of frontal headache, slight in degree, during the entire day. At 9 p.m. his temperature was 98·4°F, pulse 62.

14 December, the third day, he complained of slight frontal headache during the entire day, and was indisposed to exertion. From 6 a.m. to 6 p.m. the temperature averaged 99·2°F, and the pulse varied from 64 to 90; at 9 p.m. it was 98·4°F, the pulse 78. 15 December, the fourth day, at 6 a.m., temperature was 98·2°F, pulse 78. He still had frontal headache. At 9 a.m., temperature was 99·2°F, pulse 80; at 12 noon, the former was 99·2°F, the pulse 74. The subject now went to bed, complaining of headache and pains throughout the body. At 2 p.m., the temperature was 100°F, the pulse 80; eyes much congested; face flushed. At 6 p.m. his temperature had risen to 102°F, and the pulse to 90. He was then transferred to the yellow-fever wards. [. . .]

This case was examined by the board of experts on the 16th and 19th, and the diagnosis of yellow fever made.

[. . .] Fever subsided on 26 December, and the urine became normal on 29 December.

The period of incubation in this case, if reckoned from the time of inoculation to the hour when the patient took to his bed, was 3 days, 19½ hours.

[. . .]

It should be borne in mind that at the time when these inoculations were begun, there were only twelve non-immune residents at Camp Lazear, and that five of these were selected for experiment, viz., two in tent no. 2, and three in tent no. 5. Of these we succeeded in infecting four, viz., one in tent no. 2 and three in tent no. 5, each of whom developed an attack of yellow fever within the period of incubation of this disease. The one negative result, therefore, was in Case 2 – Moran – inoculated with a mosquito on the fifteenth day after the insect had bitten a case of yellow fever on the third day. Since this mosquito failed to infect Case 4, three days after it had bitten Moran, it follows that the result could not have been otherwise than negative in the latter case. We now know, as the result of our observations, that in the case of an insect kept at room temperature during the cool weather of November, fifteen or even eighteen days would, in all probability, be too short a time to render it capable of producing the disease.

As bearing upon the source of infection, we invite attention to the period of time during which the subjects had been kept under rigid quarantine, prior to successful inoculation, which was as follows: Case 1, fifteen days; Case 3, nine days; Case 4, nineteen days; Case 5, twenty-one days. We further desire to emphasize the fact that this epidemic of yellow fever, which affected 33·33 per cent. of the non-immune residents of Camp Lazear, did not concern the seven non-immunes occupying tents no. 1, 4, 6 and 7, *but was strictly limited to those individuals who had been bitten by contaminated mosquitoes.*

Nothing could point more forcibly to the source of this infection than the order of the occurrence of events at this camp. The precision with which the infection of the individual followed the bite of the mosquito left nothing to be desired in order to fulfill the requirements of a scientific experiment.

The epidemic having ceased on 15 December 1900, no other case of yellow fever occurred in this camp until we again began to expose individuals to inoculation. Thus fifteen days later we made the following observation:

Case 6. A Spanish immigrant, aged 27, a non-immune occupant of tent no. 6, with his full consent, was bitten at 11 a.m., 30 December 1900, by four mosquitoes – *C. fasciatus* – that had been contaminated seventeen days previously by biting a mild case of yellow fever on the first day of the disease (Case 4). These insects had been kept at a temperature of 82°F.

The subject remained in his normal condition until the evening of 2 January 1901, the third day, when he complained of frontal headache. At 6 p.m., his temperature was 99°F, pulse 64. He slept well, but still complained of headache on the following morning, 3 January. [. . .] The patient was seen by the board of experts on the second and seventh days of his attack, and the diagnosis of yellow fever confirmed.

The period of incubation in this case was 3 days, 22½ hours. The subject had remained in strict quarantine for twenty-two days preceding his inoculation.

[. . .]

In our opinion the experiments described above conclusively demonstrate that an attack of yellow fever may be readily induced in the healthy subject by the bite of mosquitoes – *C. fasciatus* – which have been previously contaminated by being fed with the blood of those sick with yellow fever, provided the insects are kept for a sufficient length of time after contamination before being applied to the person to be infected.

Our observations do not confirm Finlay's statement that the bite of the mosquito may confer an abortive attack of yellow fever, when applied to the healthy subject two to six days after it has bitten a yellow-fever patient. We have always failed to induce an attack, even of the mildest description, when we have used mosquitoes within less than twelve days from the time of contamination, although the insects were constantly kept at summer temperature. We could cite instances where we have applied mosquitoes at intervals of two, three, four, five, six, nine and eleven days following the contamination of the insect with the blood of well-marked cases of yellow fever, early in the disease, without any effect whatever being produced by the bite. Thus in one case no result followed the bite of fourteen mosquitoes which four days previously had been contaminated by biting a case of yellow fever on the first day. Again, seven days later, or eleven days after contamination, the surviving seven of these insects failed to infect an individual. On the seventeenth day after contamination, however, the bite of four of these mosquitoes – all that remained of the original fourteen – was promptly followed by an attack of yellow fever in the same individual. These insects had been kept, during the whole of this time, at an average temperature of 82°F.

Our observations would seem to indicate that after the parasite has been taken into the mosquito's stomach, a certain number of days must elapse before the insect is capable of re-conveying it to man. This period doubtless represents the time required for the parasite to pass from the insect's stomach to its salivary glands, and would appear to be about twelve days in summer weather, and most probably about eighteen or more days during the cooler winter months. It follows, also, that our observations do not confirm Finlay's opinion that the bite of the contaminated. mosquito may confer immunity against a subsequent attack of yellow fever. In our experience, an individual may be bitten on three or more occasions by contaminated mosquitoes without manifesting any symptoms of disturbance to health, and yet promptly sicken with yellow fever within a few days after being bitten by an insect capable of conveying the infection.

Acquirement of the disease

Having shown that yellow fever can be conveyed by the bite of an infected mosquito, it remains to inquire whether this disease can be acquired in any other manner. It has seemed to us that yellow fever, like the several types of malarial fever, might be induced by the injection of blood taken from the general circulation of a patient suffering with this disease. Accordingly we have subjected four individuals to this method of infection, with one negative and three positive results. Reserving the detailed description of these cases to a subsequent occasion, we may state that in one of the positive cases, an attack of pronounced yellow fever followed the subcutaneous injection of 2 cm^3 of blood taken from a vein at the bend of the elbow, on the first day of the disease, the period of incubation being three days and twenty-two hours; in the second case, 1·5 cm^3 of blood, taken on the first day of the disease, and injected in the same manner, brought about an attack within two days and twelve hours; while in our third case, the injection of

0·5 cm^3 of blood taken on the second day of the disease, produced an attack at the end of forty-one hours.

In the case mentioned as negative to the blood injection, the subsequent inoculation of this individual with mosquitoes already proved to be capable of conveying the disease, also resulted negatively. We think, therefore, that this particular individual, a Spanish immigrant, may be considered as one who probably possesses a natural immunity to yellow fever.

It is important to note that in the three cases in which the injection of the blood brought about an attack of yellow fever, careful cultures from the same blood, taken immediately after injection, failed to show the presence of Sanarelli's bacillus.

Our observations, therefore, show that the parasite of yellow fever is present in the general and capillary circulation, at least during the early stages of this disease, and that the latter may be conveyed, like the malarial parasite, either by means of the bite of the mosquito, or by the injection of blood taken from the general circulation.

Can yellow fever be propagated in any other way?

We believe that the general consensus of opinion of both the medical profession and the laity is strongly in favor of the conveyance of yellow fever by fomites. The origin of epidemics, devastating in their course, has been frequently attributed to the unpacking of trunks and boxes that contained supposedly infected clothing; and hence the efforts of health authorities, both state and national, are being constantly directed to the thorough disinfection of all clothing and bedding shipped from ports where yellow fever prevails. To such extremes have efforts at disinfection been carried, in order to prevent the importation of this disease into the United States, that, during the epidemic season, all articles of personal apparel and bedding have been subjected to disinfection, sometimes both at the port of departure and at the port of arrival; and this has been done whether the articles have previously been contaminated by contact with yellow fever patients or not. The mere fact that the individual has resided, even for a day, in a city where yellow fever is present, has been sufficient cause to subject his baggage to rigid disinfection by the sanitary authorities.

To determine, therefore, whether clothing and bedding, which have been contaminated by contact with yellow fever patients and their discharges, can convey this disease is a matter of the utmost importance. Although the literature contains many references to the failure of such contaminated articles to cause the disease, we have considered it advisable to test, by actual experiment on non-immune human beings, the theory of the conveyance of yellow fever by fomites, since we know of no other way in which this question can ever be finally determined.

For this purpose there was erected at Camp Lazear a small frame house consisting of one room 14 × 20 feet, and known as 'Building No. 1', or the 'Infected Clothing and Bedding Building'. The cubic capacity of this house was 2800 feet. It was tightly ceiled within with 'tongue and grooved' boards, and was well battened on the outside. It faced to the south and was provided with two small windows, each 26 × 34 inches in size. These windows were both placed on the south side of the building, the purpose being to prevent, as much as possible, any thorough circulation of the air within the house. They were closed by permanent wire screens of 0·5 mm mesh. In addition sliding glass sash were provided within and heavy wooden shutters without; the latter intended to prevent the entrance of sunlight into the building, as it was not deemed desirable that the disinfecting qualities of sunlight, direct or diffused, should at any time be exerted on the articles of clothing contained within this room. Entrance was effected through a small vestibule, 3 × 5 feet, also placed on the southern side of the house. This vestibule was protected without by a solid door and was divided in its middle by a wire screen door, swung on spring hinges. The inner entrance was also closed by a second wire screen door. In this way the passage of mosquitoes into this room was effectually excluded. During the day, and until after sunset, the house was kept securely closed, while by means of a suitable heating apparatus the temperature was raised to 92–5°F. Precaution was taken at the same time to maintain a sufficient humidity of the atmosphere. The average temperature of this house was thus kept at 76·2°F. for a period of sixty-three days.

On 30 November 1900, the building now being ready for occupancy, three large boxes filled with sheets, pillow-slips, blankets, etc., contaminated by contact with cases of yellow fever and their discharges were received and placed therein. The majority of the articles had been taken from the beds of patients sick with yellow fever at Las Animas Hospital, Havana, or at Columbia Barracks. Many of them had been purposely soiled with a liberal quantity of black vomit, urine and fecal matter. A dirty 'comfortable' and much-soiled pair of blankets, removed from the bed of a patient sick with yellow fever in the town of Quemados, were contained in one of these boxes. The same day, at 6 p.m., Dr R. P. Cooke, Acting Assistant-Surgeon, USA, and two privates of the hospital corps, all non-immune young Americans, entered this building and deliberately unpacked these boxes, which had been tightly closed and locked for a period of two weeks. They were careful at the same time to give each article a thorough handling and shaking in order to disseminate through the air of the room the specific agent of yellow fever, if contained in these fomites. These soiled sheets, pillowcases and blankets were used in preparing the beds in which the members of the hospital corps slept. Various soiled articles were hung around the room and placed about the bed occupied by Dr Cooke.

From this date until 19 December 1900, a series of twenty days, this room was occupied each night by these three non-immunes. Each morning the various soiled articles were carefully packed in the aforesaid boxes, and at night again unpacked and distributed about the room. During the day the residents of this house were permitted to occupy a tent pitched in the immediate vicinity, but were kept in strict quarantine.

On 12 December, a fourth box of clothing and bedding was received from Las Animas Hospital. These articles had been used on the beds of yellow-fever patients, but in addition had been purposely soiled with the bloody stools of a fatal case of this disease. As this box had been packed for a number of days, when opened and unpacked by Dr Cooke and his assistants, on 12 December, the odor was so offensive as to compel them to retreat from the house. They pluckily returned, however, within a short time and spent the night as usual.

On 19 December, these three non-immunes were placed in quarantine for five days and then given the liberty of the camp.

All had remained in perfect health, notwithstanding their stay of twenty nights amid such unwholesome surroundings.

During the week 20–27 December, the following articles were also placed in this house, viz.: pajamas suits, 1; undershirts, 2; night-shirts, 4; pillow-slips, 4; sheets, 6; blankets, 5; pillows, 2; mattresses, 1. These articles had been removed from the persons and beds of four patients sick with yellow fever and were very much soiled, as any change of clothing or bed-linen during their attacks had been purposely avoided, the object being to obtain articles as thoroughly contaminated as possible.

From 21 December 1900, till 10 January 1901, this building was again occupied by two non-immune young Americans, under the same conditions as the preceding occupants, except that these men slept every night in the very garments worn by yellow fever patients throughout their entire attacks, besides making use exclusively of their much-soiled pillow-slips, sheets and blankets. At the end of twenty-one nights of such intimate contact with these fomites, they also went into quarantine, from which they were released five days later in perfect health.

From 11 January till 31 January, a period of twenty days, 'Building No. 1' continued to be occupied by two other non-immune Americans, who, like those who preceded them, have slept every night in the beds formerly occupied by yellow fever patients and in the night-shirts used by these patients throughout the attack, without change. In addition, during the last fourteen nights of their occupancy of this house they have slept, each night, with their pillows covered with towels that had been thoroughly soiled with the blood drawn from both the general and capillary circulation, on the first day of the disease, in the case of a well-marked attack of yellow fever. Notwithstanding this trying ordeal, these men have continued to remain in perfect health.

The attempt which we have therefore made to infect 'Building No. 1', and its seven non-immune occupants, during a period of sixty-three days, has proved an absolute failure. [. . .]

The question here naturally arises: How does a house become infected with yellow fever? This we have attempted to solve by the erection at Camp Lazear of a second house, known as 'Building No. 2', or the 'Infected Mosquito Building'. This was in all respects similar to 'Building No. 1', except that the door and windows were placed on opposite sides of the building so as to give through-and-through ventilation. It was divided, also, by a wire-screen partition, extending from floor to ceiling, into two rooms, 12 × 14 feet and 8 × 14 feet respectively. Whereas, all articles admitted to 'Building No. 1' had been soiled by contact with yellow-fever patients, all articles admitted to 'Building No. 2' were first carefully disinfected by steam before being placed therein.

On 21 December 1900, at 11.45 a.m., there were set free in the larger room of this building fifteen mosquitoes – *C. fasciatus* – which had previously been contaminated by biting yellow-fever patients, as follows: one, a severe case, on the second day, 27 November 1900, twenty-four days; three, a well-marked case, on the first day, 9 December 1900, twelve days; four, a mild case, on the first day, 13 December 1900, eight days; seven, a well-marked case on the first day, 16 December 1900, five days – total, fifteen.

Only one of these insects was considered capable of conveying the infection, viz., the mosquito that had bitten a severe case twenty-four days before; while three others – the twelve-day insects – had possibly reached the dangerous stage, as they had been kept at an average temperature of 82°F.

At 12 noon of the same day, John J. Moran – already referred to as Case 2 in this report – a non-immune American, entered the room where the mosquitoes had been freed, and remained thirty minutes. During this time he was bitten about the face and hands by several insects. At 4.30 p.m., the same day, he again entered and remained twenty minutes, and was again bitten. The following day, at 4.30 p.m., he, for the third time, entered the room, and was again bitten.

Case 7. On 25 December 1900, at 6 a.m., the fourth day, Moran complained of slight dizziness and frontal headache. At 11 a.m. he went to bed, complaining of increased headache and malaise, with a temperature of 99·6°F, pulse 88; at noon the temperature was 100·4°F, the pulse 98; at 1 p.m., 101·2°F, the pulse 96, and his eyes were much injected and face suffused. He was removed to the yellow-fever wards. He was seen on several occasions by the board of experts and the diagnosis of yellow fever confirmed.

The period of incubation in this case, dating from the first visit to 'Building No. 2', was three days and twenty-three hours. If reckoned from his last visit it was two days and eighteen hours.

There was no other possible source for his infection, as he had been strictly quarantined at Camp Lazear for a period of thirty-two days prior to his exposure in the mosquito building.

During each of Moran's visits, two non-immunes remained in this same building, only protected from the mosquitoes by the wire-screen partition. From 21 December 1900, till 8 January 1901, inclusive – eighteen nights – these non-immunes have slept in this house, only protected by the wire screen partition. These men have remained in perfect health to the present time.

On 28 December, after an interval of seven days, this house was again entered by a non-immune American, who remained twenty-five minutes. The subject was bitten by only one insect. The following day he again entered and remained fifteen minutes, and was again bitten by one mosquito. The result of these two visits was entirely negative. As the mortality among the insects in this room, from some unknown cause, had been surprisingly large, it is possible that the subject was bitten by insects not more than thirteen days old, in which case they would probably not infect, since they had been kept for only five days at a temperature of 82°F, and for eight days at the mean temperature of the room, 78°F.

Be this as it may, nothing can be more striking or instructive as bearing upon the cause of house infection in yellow fever, than when we contrast the results obtained in our attempts to infect Buildings No. 1 and No. 2; for whereas, in the former *all* of seven non-immunes escaped the infection, although exposed to the most intimate contact with the fomites for an average period of twenty-one nights each; in the latter, an exposure, reckoned by as many minutes, was quite sufficient to give an attack of yellow fever to one out of two persons who entered the building – 50 per cent.

Thus at Camp Lazear, of seven non-immunes whom we attempted to infect by means of the bites of contaminated mosquitoes, we have succeeded in conveying the disease to six, or 85·71 per cent. On the other hand, seven non-immunes whom we tried to infect by means of fomites, under particularly favorable circumstances, we did not succeed in a single instance. Out of a total of eighteen non-immunes whom we have inoculated with contaminated mosquitoes, since we began this line of investigation, eight, or 44·4 per cent, have contracted yellow fever. If we exclude those individuals bitten by mosquitoes that had been kept less than twelve days after contamination, and which were, therefore, probably incapable of conveying the disease, we have to record eight positive and two negative results – 80 per cent.

Conclusions

1. The mosquito – *C. fasciatus* – serves as the intermediate host for the parasite of yellow fever.

2. Yellow fever is transmitted to the non-immune individual by means of the bite of the mosquito that has previously fed on the blood of those sick with this disease.

3. An interval of about twelve days or more after contamination appears to be necessary before the mosquito is capable of conveying the infection.

4. The bite of the mosquito at an earlier period after contamination does not appear to confer any immunity against a subsequent attack.

5. Yellow fever can also be experimentally produced by the subcutaneous injection of blood taken from the general circulation during the first and second days of this disease.

6. An attack of yellow fever, produced by the bite of the mosquito, confers immunity against the subsequent injection of the blood of an individual suffering from the non-experimental form of this disease.

7. The period of incubation in thirteen cases of experimental yellow fever has varied from forty-one hours to five days and seventeen hours.

8. Yellow fever is not conveyed by fomites, and hence disinfection of articles of clothing, bedding, or merchandise, supposedly contaminated by contact with those sick with this disease, is unnecessary.

9. A house may be said to be infected with yellow fever only when there are present within its walls contaminated mosquitoes capable of conveying the parasite of this disease.

10. The spread of yellow fever can be most effectually controlled by measures directed to the destruction of mosquitoes and the protection of the sick against the bites of these insects.

11. While the mode of propagation of yellow fever has now been definitely determined, the specific cause of this disease remains to be discovered.

F. G. Banting and C. H. Best

The discovery of insulin illustrates the cooperative nature of science and the way that many different observations that had long seemed isolated can eventually fall into a pattern. The story of the discovery of insulin illustrates the way a pattern gradually gets established, and the impetus that results when the right man investigates at the right time and in the right place.

Diabetes had for centuries been a well-recognized clinical entity, but the relevant causal factors were completely unknown. In the last half of the nineteenth century progress was made towards understanding the disease. Claude Bernard provided the basic principles of glucose metabolism. Physiological researches clarified the idea of 'internal secretion', where glandular products enter into the blood stream directly, in contrast to those products which are 'excreted' into a duct and conveyed to the outside world or to other organs. Anatomical researches on the pancreas indicated a dual nature of that gland, with two types of tissue – acinar structures that have an excretory duct and so-called islet tissue that discharges its secretion directly into the blood stream. Mering and Minkowsky furnished an important step when they produced diabetes in dogs by removing the pancreas – a feat of great technical virtuosity at that time. Evidence accumulated that diabetes was connected with the islet tissue which, when normal, seemed to produce an 'anti-diabetic' substance connected with sugar metabolism.

If this substance were absent in diabetics, perhaps a suitable extract of normal pancreas would provide a substitute, whereby the disease might be effectively treated. But extracts of whole pancrea proved unsatisfactory, for in the process of preparation digestive agents arising from the acinar tissue destroyed the anti-diabetic principle. How could this agent be eliminated?

Previous work had suggested that the acinar tissue would atrophy and eventually disappear if the excretory duct of the pancreas were ligated. The islet tissue, discharging its anti-diabetic secretions directly into the blood, would remain intact.

A 'degenerated' pancreas, lacking acinar tissue, might thus serve as the source of the extract.

But how could one tell if an extract contained the anti-diabetic principle, and make any sort of quantitative comparisons? Dogs made diabetic by total excision of the pancreas might serve as a suitable model. Extracts could then be tested by administration to such an animal.

Banting, working in MacLeod's laboratory, had brought all these various threads together. He not only conceived a hypothesis, but with precise and critical experimentation he (with the assistance of Best and others) was able to establish it as a fact and prove its validity. His experiments opened the way for modern treatment of diabetes.

Banting's achievement was possible only after various techniques had advanced to a high degree. Modern histology had distinguished the various components of the pancreas, while physiology had determined the relative functions. Anaesthesia and asepsis made complicated experimental surgery possible. Biochemistry had reached a high development, to provide techniques of extraction and also of analysis, to determine blood and urine components with precision.

The paper which is excerpted here gives the background, reasoning and the experimental methods and proofs. It represents the two significant components of modern science – the clear thinking and critical acumen that we find in scientist-physicians throughout history; and the accumulation of factual knowledge and technical procedures that permitted both the formulation of a hypothesis and its actual demonstration.

23 The Internal Secretions of the Pancreas (1922)

Excerpts from F. G. Banting and C. H. Best, 'The Internal Secretion of the Pancreas', *Journal of Laboratory and Clinical Medicine*, vol. 7, February 1922, pp. 251–66.

The hypothesis underlying this series of experiments was first formulated by one of us in November 1920, while reading an article dealing with the relation of the islets of Langerhans to diabetes. From the passage in this article, which gives a résumé of degenerative changes in the acini of the pancreas following ligation of the ducts, the idea presented itself that since the acinous, but not the islet tissue, degenerates after this operation, advantage might be taken of this fact to prepare an active extract of islet tissue. The subsidiary hypothesis was that trypsinogen or its derivatives was antagonistic to the internal secretion of the gland. The failures of other investigators in this much-worked field were thus accounted for.

The feasibility of the hypothesis having been recognized by Professor J. J. R. Macleod, work was begun under his direction in May 1921, in the Physiological Laboratory of the University of Toronto.

In this paper no attempt is made to give a complete review of the literature. A short résumé, however, of some of the outstanding articles which tend to attribute to the islets of Langerhans the control of carbohydrate metabolism, is submitted.

In 1889 Mering and Minkowski found that total pancreatectomy in dogs resulted in severe and fatal diabetes. Following this, many different observers experimented with animals of various species and found in all types examined, a glycosuria and fatal cachexia after this operation. The fact was thus established that the pancreas was responsible for this form of diabetes. In 1884, Arnozan and Vaillard had ligated the pancreatic ducts in rabbits and found that within twenty-four hours the ducts become dilated; the epithelial cells begin to desquamate; and that there are protoplasmic changes in the acinous cells. On the seventh day there is a beginning of round-celled infiltration. On the fourteenth day the parenchyma was mostly replaced by fibrous tissue.

Sscobolew in 1902 noted in addition to the above, that there was a gradual atrophy and sclerosis of the pancreas with no glucosuria. However, in the later stages, from thirty to one hundred and twenty days after ligation of the ducts, he found involvement of the islets and accompanying glucosuria.

[. . .]

W. G. MacCallum, in 1909, ligated the ducts draining the tail third of the pancreas. After seven months he excised the remaining two-thirds. This was followed by a mild glucosuria. Three weeks later he removed the degenerated tail third. This second operation resulted in an extreme and fatal glucosuria. Kirkbridge, in 1912, repeated and corroborated MacCallum's findings and, by the use of Lane's method of staining, proved that the atrophic tissue contained healthy islets.

Kamimura in 1917, working on rabbits, traced the degenerative changes in the parenchymatous tissue of the pancreas after ligation of the ducts, and found that the islets remained normal and that the animal did not develop glucosuria as long as the islets were left intact.

The first attempt to ulilize the pancreas in defects of carbohydrate metabolism was made by Minkowski. This worker tried the effect of pancreatic feeding, with no beneficial results. Up to the present time only useless or even harmful effects have been obtained from repeated attempts to use this method.

[. . .]

Murlin prepared an alkaline extract of pancreatic tissue and after injection of this solution, secured a reduction in sugar excreted in a diabetic animal. Kleiner has pointed out that the reduction secured by Murlin might be due to the alkali *per se*. Kleiner himself has shown that 'unfiltered-water extracts of fresh pancreas diluted with 0·90 per cent NaCl when administered slowly usually resulted in a marked decrease in blood sugar.' There was no compensating increase in urine sugar, but rather a decrease, which Kleiner suggests may be partly due to a temporary toxic renal effect. Hemoglobin estimations made during the experiment showed that the reduction in blood sugar was not a dilution phenomenon. [. . .]

From the work of the above-mentioned observers we may conclude: (1) that the secretion produced by the acinous cells of the pancreas are in no way connected with carbohydrate utilization; (2) that all injections of whole-gland extract have been futile as a therapeutic measure in defects of carbohydrate utilization; (3) that the islets of Langerhans are essential in the control of carbohydrate metabolism. According to Macleod there are two possible mechanisms by which the islets might accomplish this control: (1) the blood might be modified while passing through the islet tissue, i.e., the islets might be detoxicating stations, and (2) the islets might produce an internal secretion.

We submit the following experiments which we believe give convincing evidence that it is this latter mechanism which is in operation.

[. . .]

Methods

The first chart [all charts are omitted] is a record of an animal depancreatized by the Hédon method. The details of this operation are given in Hédon's article. The remaining records are of animals (females) completely depancreatized at the initial operation. The procedure is as follows: [here follows the technique of the operation to produce diabetic animals].

We have found that animals between eight and sixteen months old are the most suitable for this operation. At this age the pancreas is not so firmly fixed as it becomes later.

We first ligated, under general anesthesia, the pancreatic ducts in a number of dogs. (Blood sugar estimations on these animals were recorded from time to time. We have no record of a hyperglycemia.)

The extract was prepared as follows: The dog was given a lethal dose of chloroform. The degenerated pancreas was swiftly removed and sliced into a chilled mortar containing Ringer's solution. The mortar was placed in freezing mixture and the contents partially frozen. The half frozen gland was then completely macerated. The solution was filtered through paper and the filtrate, having been raised to body temperature, was injected intravenously.

[. . .]

We performed several experiments with the object of exhausting the zymogen granules of the pancreas. Prolonged secretin injections and vagus stimulation below the diaphragm were practiced. Fortune favored us in the first experiment. In subsequent attempts we were never able to exhaust the gland sufficiently to obtain an extract free from the disturbing effects of some constituent of pancreatic juice.

[. . .] We find the average normal blood sugar, from observations on thirty normal dogs, to be 0·090 per cent.

[. . .]

Results

Chart 1 contains the record of a 6·5 kg dog (410). This experiment is not conclusive but is interesting to us at least, since we administered the first dose of extract of degenerated pancreas to this animal. On 11 July, the pancreas, with the exception of the processus uncinatus, was removed. [. . .] The animal continued to lose weight and seemed to be entering the cachexial condition characteristic of depancreatized, animals which had become infected.

[. . .]

At 10 a.m. 30 July, the percentage of blood sugar was 0·20; 4 cm^3 of extract of degenerated pancreas were injected intravenously. At 11 a.m. the blood sugar had fallen to 0·12 per cent. The injections of extract are shown in the chart. At 12 a.m. 20 g of sugar in 200 cm^3 of water were given by stomach tube.

The obvious criticism of this experiment is that the animal was moribund when the effect of the extract was tried. The interesting features, which gave us great encouragement are (1) the extract caused a sudden fall in the blood sugar and (2) that in the presence of the extract the animal excreted 0·21 g of a 20 g injection in a period of five hours following the injection, in contrast to an excretion of 15·88 g of a 25 g injection in the same interval, when no extract was administered.

Chart 2 is the record of dog 92, weight 11·9 kg. A complete pancreatectomy was performed on this animal at 3 p.m. 11 August. The first injection of extract was given six hours after the operation and subsequently an injection every four hours. This extract was freshly prepared from a 10 kg dog whose pancreatic ducts had been ligated for ten weeks. One hundred and twenty-five cubic centimetres of extract were prepared from the gland residue but this supply was exhaused by 2 p.m., 13 August, after which other extracts were used. Blood samples were always taken before the injections of extract.

On 12 August, the blood sugar curve shows that neither 5 cm³ nor 8 cm³ of this extract every four hours were sufficient to counterbalance the upward trend of the percentage of sugar of the blood. At 10 p.m. the dose was increased to 12 cm³ and a marked fall is noted. The chart at 10 a.m. 14 August records the reduction of the percentage of sugar in the blood below its normal level, as a result of extract from another degenerated gland. [. . .]

On 16 and 17 August effects of extracts from normal glands were tested. A normal pancreas from a 10 kg animal was divided into three equal parts. One third was extracted with neutral saline, the second portion with 0·1 per cent HCl and the third with 0·1 per cent NaOH. On 17 August at 4 p.m. the neutral whole gland extract was administered. A marked fall in blood sugar resulted. The acid and alkaline extracts were injected at 12 p.m. 17 August, and 7 a.m. 18 August. The last two injections were perhaps not given a fair opportunity to develop their effects. We do not take colorimeter readings by artificial light and therefore did not have an accurate knowledge of the height of blood sugar at these times.

The conclusion from this experiment is that freshly prepared neutral or acid extracts of the whole pancreas do have a reducing effect on blood sugar, thus confirming Kleiner. It may be stated here that repeated injections of whole gland extracts cause marked thrombosis of the veins where the injections are made and a noticeable interference with kidney function. It is obvious from the chart that the whole gland extract is much weaker than that from the degenerated gland.

[. . .]

Chart 3 is the record of dog 408. The weight of this animal was 9 kg. The details of the experiment will be given rather fully.

The normal blood sugar of dog 408 was 0·090 per cent. Eighteen hours after pancreatectomy the percentage of sugar in the blood was 0·27. Twenty-two hours after the operation, 1 p.m. 4 August, the blood sugar was 0·26 per cent. During the twenty-two hours 3·10 g of sugar were excreted. The volume of urine was 494 cm³. At 1 p.m. we administered 5 cm³ of extract of degenerated pancreas which had been prepared four days previously and kept in cold storage. At 2 p.m. the blood sugar was 0·16 per cent. At 3 p.m. the percentage of sugar in the blood had fallen to 0·15. From 1 to 3 p.m. 0·19 g of sugar were excreted in a volume of 26 cm³ of urine. [. . .] From 3 p.m. to 7 p.m. the percentage of sugar in the blood shows a gradual rise from 0·15 to 0·25 per cent. This latter level was maintained until 9 p.m. The chart shows a slight rise in sugar excretion following the rise of blood sugar. At 9 p.m. 5 cm³ of extract which had been exposed to room temperature for one hour was injected intravenously. The blood sugar was reduced to a value of 0·18 per cent. The chart shows a gradual ascent from this value to 0·27 per cent. At 10 p.m. the percentage of sugar in the blood was 0·27 At this hour 5 cm³ of extract of liver, prepared in precisely the same manner as the pancreatic extract, were administered intravenously One hour later the blood sugar was 0·30 per cent. This level was maintained during the following three hours. It was unaffected by an injection of 5 cm³ of extract of spleen. [. . .] At 2 p.m. (b. s. 0·3 per cent), 5 cm³ of an extract of degenerated pancreas were injected. A sharp fall in the blood sugar resulted. At 3 p.m. and again at 4 p.m. a similar dose of extract was given. The chart records the lasting effect. The 2 p.m. level of 0·30 per cent was regained twelve hours after the first injection. The hourly excretion of sugar ran approximately parallel with the percentage of sugar in the blood. Between 1 p.m. and 2 p.m. 0·52 g were excreted. Less than 0·02 g were excreted between 7 p.m. and 8 p.m. [. . .] At twelve noon 6 August the percentage sugar in the blood was 0·40 per cent. Five cubic centimetres of boiled extract of degenerated pancreas was injected intravenously at this stage and caused no reduction of blood sugar. At 12 midnight 6 August 5 cm³ of extract of degenerated pancreas which had been prepared 48 h previously were administered. The blood sugar fell from 0·43 per cent at 12 p.m. to 0·37 per cent at 1 a.m. Five cubic centimetres doses were given at 1, 2 and 3 a.m. and a 25 cm³ dose at 4 a.m. The chart shows the reduction in blood sugar to a normal level and the beginning of an upward trend five hours after the last injection of extract. The animal died at 12 a.m. 7 August.

A brief description of the clinical condition of the animal at various stages of the experiment is necessary for the correct interpretation of the above results. The animal made a good post-operative recovery and was able to retain water and meat after the second day following the operation. On the morning of 5 August we noticed that the condition of the animal was much worse. It appeared excessively tired, did not eat, and vomited after drinking water and also after extract of spleen given intravenously. At 5 p.m. 5 August the animal appeared considerably improved. It retained water and ate meat. On 6 August at 10 p.m. the abdominal wound was moist with exudate, and the animal was not so active as on the preceding day. No marked variation from this condition was observed until 4 a.m. when 25 cm³ of extract were administered. After this injection the animal had a marked reaction and appeared to be dying. It was revived slightly by intravenous and intraperitoneal injections of warm saline. Considerable improvement was noted at 7 a.m.; the dog was able to stand. The improvement was short-lived. The dog died at 12 a.m. 7 August. The post-mortem showed a widespread abdominal infection. There was no sign of pancreatic tissue.

The entire degenerated pancreas from one 8 kg dog and approximately one-half the degenerated gland from a 6 kg dog was the substrate of the extract used in this experiment.

Chart 4, dog 9, gives additional evidence on several important points which have been referred to previously. At 6 p.m. 8 September, we administered 10 cm³ of extract of degenerated pancreas *per rectum*. There was no reduction in blood sugar at 7 p.m. when we gave 12 cm³ of extract of exhausted gland intravenously. The chart records the effect of this and subsequent injections of the same material. At 6 a.m., 10 September, we administered 15 cm³ of extract of exhausted gland *per rectum*. There was no effect. At 8 a.m. 10 September, 15 cm³ of extract of exhausted gland were injected intravenously. The drop in blood sugar was very marked [from 300 to 130]. Twenty cubic centimetres of exhausted gland extract, made 1 per cent alkaline with NaOH, were incubated three hours at body temperature with 10 cm³ of active pancreatic juice. This solution was neutralized and injected intravenously at 7 p.m. 10 September. No reduction in blood sugar resulted. At 2 p.m. 11 September, 20 cm³ of acid extract incubated for three hours at 37·5°F. were injected. The curve shows the drop in blood sugar [of about 100 mg]. On 13 September, at 9 a.m. and 2 p.m. the effect of extracts from the partially exhausted gland of a cat is shown [about 75 mg drop each time]. This extract produces a pronounced general reaction.

We observe that extracts prepared from these more or less exhausted glands, while retaining to some extent the reducing effect upon blood and urine sugar, produce many symptoms of toxicity which are absent after injections of extracts from completely degenerated glands.

[The authors then describe an experiment to prove that the reduction in blood sugar is not a dilution effect.]

Chart 6 is the record of a short, but very interesting experiment which again demonstrates the remarkable effect of the extract of degenerated pancreas upon the power of a diabetic animal to retain sugar. At 11 a.m. on 8 November (b.s. 0·35 per cent), 10 g of sugar were injected intravenously. The curve shows the rise in blood sugar [to 0·40]. In the four hours following the injection, 10·88 g of sugar were excreted. From 3 to 9 p.m. 78 cm³ of dilute extract were injected in 13 cm³ doses. At 9 p.m. (b.s. 0·09 per cent), 10 g of sugar were injected. The curve shows the effect on blood sugar [to 0·23] and sugar excretion. The effect of partially degenerated gland extract, five weeks after ligation of the ducts, upon the kidneys is shown here. This extract may produce a raised threshold to sugar or a condition of anuria, as in this experiment.

In the course of our experiments we have administered over seventy-five doses of extract from degenerated pancreatic tissue to ten different diabetic animals. Since the extract has always produced a reduction of the percentage sugar of the blood and of the sugar excreted in the urine, we feel justified in stating that this extract contains the internal secretion of the pancreas. Some of our more recent experiments, which are not yet completed, give, in addition to still more conclusive evidence regarding the sugar retaining power of diabetic animals treated with extract, some interesting facts regarding the chemical nature of the active principle of the internal secretion. These results, together with a study of the respiratory exchange in diabetic animals before and after administration of extract, will be reported in a subsequent communication.

We have always observed a distinct improvement in the clinical condition of diabetic dogs after administration of extract of degenerated pancreas, but it is very obvious that the results of our experimental work, as reported in this paper do not at present justify the therapeutic administration of degenerated gland extracts to cases of diabetes mellitus in the clinic.

Conclusions

The results of the experimental work reported in this article may be summarized as follows:

Intravenous injections of extract from dog's pancreas, removed from seven to ten weeks after ligation of the ducts, invariably exercises a reducing influence upon the percentage sugar of the blood and the amount of sugar excreted in the urine.

Rectal injections are not effective.

The extent and duration of the reduction varies directly with the amount of extract injected.

Pancreatic juice destroys the active principle of the extract.

That the reducing action is not a dilution phenomenon is indicated by the following facts: (1) hemoglobin estimations before and after administration of extract are identical; (2) injections of large quantities of saline do not effect the blood sugar; (3) similar quantities of extracts of other tissues do not cause a reduction of blood sugar.

Extract made 0·1 per cent acid is effectual in lowering the blood sugar.

The presence of extract enables a diabetic animal to retain a much greater percentage of injected sugar than it would otherwise.

Extract prepared in neutral saline and kept in cold storage retains its potency for at least seven days.

Boiled extract has no effect on the reduction of blood sugar.

Norman Simon and John Harley

Modern medicine has analytical tools which permit physicians to make extraordinarily fine analyses and discriminations. These comprise the so-called 'tests', whose glamour captivates both laymen and physician. But 'tests' by themselves, no matter how delicate, are not 'scientific'. More important is the critical judgment which sees the need for tests, and can interpret the results. The brief case report given here throws light on that critical judgment which is the core of 'scientific' medicine.

Nature manifests itself in patterns, and if the physician, trying to make a diagnosis, can identify part of the pattern, he may jump to conclusions and believe that he has the entire pattern. But there is scope for error. Similarities in some respects may mislead the physician and cause him to neglect differences. Actually, the differences might be more significant, and proper attention to these differences would lead to a quite different diagnosis.

The present case concerns a woman who suffered from a localized skin lesion that developed under her wedding ring. Several physicians whom she consulted considered it a 'contact dermatitis', that is, sensitivity to some product with which she came into contact. The most likely agent seemed to be a detergent used in dishwashing. Although she kept her hands away from detergents, the lesion did not fully clear up.

The patient's husband, a professor of engineering, also suffered from an apparently similar dermatitis under his wedding ring. He did not believe the physicians' diagnosis, but thought the entire disease might depend on some quite different set of circumstances. There occurred to him the possibility of radiation effect. This represented only a hypothesis, but one which could be subjected to tests. With appropriate apparatus, the rings were examined and found in fact to be radioactive.

Now the diagnosis of contact dermatitis, implying an allergic causation, had a great deal to recommend it, for there were certain similarities between this particular illness and other examples of proven skin sensitivities. But unfortunately, the physicians paid insufficient attention to one important feature: *the diagnosis*, contact dermatitis, *was not adequately verified*. Eliminating the presumed causal agents did not remedy the condition. The patient's husband finally became convinced that this failure invalidated the diagnosis, and he sought some other alternative. His insistence led to the diagnosis of radiation dermatitis, quite distinct from contact dermatitis.

The important feature here is the perception that the evidence for contact dermatitis was not adequate to support that diagnosis. Once this was perceived, the scientific investigator sought new evidence, and utilized a highly sophisticated tool – the Geiger counter – to secure it. The new data quickly led to a different diagnosis, radiation dermatitis. No one thought of it until the scientist – the husband – uncovered new data which pointed to it.

This is the prototype of scientific progress in medicine. *Someone perceives a lack of congruence between an assertion (diagnosis) and the actual course of events*. This perception, if deeply felt, leads to further search. Someone who realizes that the available evidence simply isn't good enough seeks for more and better evidence. Progress depends on the insight of particular individuals who 'see' and pay attention to discrepancies, while their less gifted colleagues fail to see or else ignore what they have seen.

Scientific medicine comprises an attitude, an attitude toward evidence, and has no necessary connection with techniques, apparatus or quantitation. These can make a brave show but without critical judgment are quite insignificant.

24 Skin Reactions from Gold Jewelry Contaminated with Radon Deposit (1967)

Excerpts from N. Simon and J. Harley, 'Skin reactions from gold jewelry contaminated with radon deposit', *Journal of the American Medical Association*, vol. 200, April 1967, pp. 254–5.

Gold jewelry may be contaminated sufficiently with radiation to represent a hazard to the wearer. The finding of gold rings containing decay products of radon has prompted this report.

Report of cases

A professor and his wife were seen by us because of chronic skin lesions of their ring fingers and the recent finding of radioactivity in their wedding rings. In December 1940, twenty-six years ago, they were married in a double-ring ceremony. They wore their rings constantly, and the bride noticed a rash under her ring after about a year. Subsequently a skin reaction also developed under the husband's ring. In those early years of their marriage they were living in Indiana, and the skin rashes were considered to be due to detergents which had just been available to the housewife. The itching, redness, and later blistering of the fingers finally forced both husband and wife to remove their rings permanently in 1945, about five years after their wedding. For the past twenty years or so, the wife has been wearing a cotton glove under a rubber glove whenever she washes dishes, since her lesion still appeared to be a contact dermatitis to the numerous physicians who saw her over the period of years. Her lesion was so resistant to any therapy that even X-ray treatments were administered by dermatologists in 1951 and again in 1953. The wife considers her finger to be in relatively good condition at the present time, but there is an irregularly bordered, raised thickening of the skin encircling the base of the left ring finger with smaller, scaling 'kissing' lesions of the adjacent fingers. The underlying phalanges are normal on X-ray film. Also, the subcutaneous tissue moves readily over the bone.

Her husband has deep fissures surrounded by keratotic, dry, raised skin, particulary on the volar aspect of his left ring finger. The 'irritation' of his finger is worse during the summer when he gardens and goes boating. An X-ray examination of his involved finger also shows normal underlying bone. The skin moves freely over the bone, and there is no indication of deep fibrosis. In the left axilla there is a 1 cm, ovoid, soft, palpable lymph node. The lesion in the husband's finger was suggestive of tumor, but both patients were advised to have excision of the involved skin with grafting of the defect.

Memorial Hospital ring

Another radioactive gold ring had been retained in a shielded container in the Department of Medical Physics of the Memorial Hospital in New York city. Edith Quimby, PhD, professor emeritus of Radiation Physics at the Columbia College of Physicians and Surgeons, recalled that more than thirty years ago a gold ring was made from tiny pieces of gold tubing which had contained radon made by the radon plant which was designed by the late Giacchino Failla, PhD, for Memorial Hospital for Cancer and Allied Diseases in New York. When a skin reaction developed in the finger under the ring, the ring was removed and placed in storage. The gold in this ring was recorded to contain more than 100 decayed radon seeds.

Comment

How were the wedding rings determined to be radioactive? The husband, a university professor of engineering, became sceptical about the explanations given him for the cause of the skin lesion on his wife's and his own ring fingers. Numerous physicians during a score of years had attributed the skin reaction to contact with detergents and other dish-washing preparations. Even if this was an acceptable explanation for his wife's reaction, he used other soaps and washed no dishes and had a similar reaction. Quite serendipitously he thought the reaction might be due to radiation. He gave the rings to a colleague at his university who established the presence of radioactivity with a Geiger–Muller tube.

Analysis of the rings indicates the activity to be due to the decay products of radon, radium D and E, emitters of beta radiation with a long half-life of more than twenty years.

Radon-222, an inert gas, is a daughter element of radium-226. The gas is compressed into a tiny gold tube or seed for use in implantation of tumors. Radium D or lead-210 and radium E or bismuth-210 are the important decay products of radon which deposit on gold and which may remain active enough to cause superficial skin reactions for many years. The gold of the wedding rings and of the Memorial Hospital ring contained decayed radon seeds or gold tubing containing unused and decayed radon from a radon plant. Further, the gold had not been refined; during this process the radon deposit would have been separated.

Some industrial refiners of gold test each batch for radioactivity before processing, and one local company has detected such a radon-contaminated batch as recently as a few years ago. But all gold handlers are not equipped to detect radiation, and it is reasonable to assume that contaminated gold has escaped into the jewelry market. This assumption warrants investigation into observations made by jewelers that some people can wear one type of gold, but another 'type' irritates the skin.

Several decades ago there was mention of the possibility of the inadvertent use of gold seeds of decayed radon in dental appliances. Like a wedding ring, a gold dental appliance is usually worn constantly, and its contamination could result in a significant buccal reaction. We have not actually seen an oral reaction to such contaminated gold.

Conclusion

When unexplained skin reaction results from contact with gold jewelry, radiation reaction should be suspected, and the gold should be tested for radioactivity. Gold to be processed for jewelry and dental use should be monitored for radiation contamination with gold seeds of decayed radon.

Further Reading

These suggestions for further reading do not pretend to any coverage of medical history, nor do they represent any sort of scholarly bibliography. The items listed have to do with the points of view expressed in the excerpts and the expository material, and are chosen to provide the reader the barest introduction to the riches that await him. I have restricted the list to some secondary sources in English. No primary-source material, no journal articles, and no works in foreign languages are included.

General

E. H. Ackerknecht, *A Short History of Medicine*, Ronald Press, 1955.

A. Castiglioni, *A History of Medicine* (translated by E. B. Krumbhaar), 2nd edn, Knopf, 1947.

D. Guthrie, *A History of Medicine*, Nelson, 1958.

L. S. King, *Growth of Medical Thought*, University of Chicago Press, 1963.

G. Rosen, *A History of Public Health*, MD Publications, 1958.

C. Singer, and E. A. Underwood, *A Short History of Medicine*, 2nd edn, Oxford University Press, 1962.

Part One – The Classical Heritage

T. C. Allbutt, *Greek Medicine in Rome*, Macmillan, 1921.

B. Farrington, *Greek Science: Its Meaning for Us*, Penguin, 1953.

W. A. Heidel, *Hippocratic Medicine, Its Spirit and Method*, Columbia University Press, 1941.

H. D. F. Kitto, *The Greeks*, Penguin, 1959.

R. E. Siegel, *Galen's Systems of Physiology and Medicine*, S. Karger, 1968.

Part Two – Revolt

K. D. Keele, *William Harvey: The Man, the Physician, and the Scientist*, Nelson, 1965.

G. Keynes, *The Life of William Harvey*, Clarendon Press, 1966.

L. S. King, *Growth of Medical Thought*, University of Chicago Press, 1963, pp. 86–174.

C. D. O'Malley, *Andreas Vesalius of Brussels 1514–1564*, University of California Press, 1964.

W. Pagel, *Paracelsus: An Introduction to Philosophical Medicine in the Era of the Renaissance*, S. Karger, 1958.

W. Pagel, *William Harvey's Biological Ideas: Selected Aspects and Historical Background*, Hafner, 1967.

Part Three – Development

E. Ackerknecht, *Medicine at the Paris Hospital, 1794–1848*, Johns Hopkins Press, 1967.

J. R. Baker, *Abraham Trembley, Scientist and Philosopher 1710–1784*, Edward Arnold, 1952.

I. S. Cutter, and H. R. Viets, *A Short History of Midwifery*, Saunders, 1964.

M. Foster, *Lectures on the History of Physiology during the Sixteenth, Seventeenth and Eighteenth Centuries*, Cambridge University Press, 1901.

S. R. Gloyne, *John Hunter*, Livingstone, 1950.

L. S. King, *Medical World of the Eighteenth Century*, University of Chicago Press, 1958.

L. S. King, *The Road to Medical Enlightenment, 1650–1695*, Macdonald, 1970.

J. Kobler, *The Reluctant Surgeon: A Biography of John Hunter*, Doubleday, 1960.

G. A. Lindeboom, *Herman Boerhaave, The Man and His Work*, Methuen, 1968.

M. Ornstein, *The Role of Scientific Societies in the Seventeenth Century*, University of Chicago Press, 1928.

S. Paget, *John Hunter, Man of Science and Surgeon (1728–1793)*, Fisher Unwin, 1897.

W. Radcliffe, *Milestones in Midwifery*, John Wright, 1967.

J. Thomson, *An Account of the Life, Lectures, and Writings of William Cullen, M.D.*, Blackwood, 1859.

A. Vartanian, *La Mettrie's 'L'Homme Machine': A Study in the Origins of an Idea*, Princeton University Press, 1960.

A. Wolf, *A History of Science, Technology, and Philosophy in the Eighteenth Century*, new edition prepared by Douglas McKie, Allen & Unwin, 2nd edn, 1952.

A. Wolf, *A History of Science, Technology, and Philosophy in the Sixteenth and Seventeenth Centuries*, new edition prepared by Douglas McKie, Allen & Unwin, 2nd edn, 1950.

Part Four – Fruition

E. H. Ackerknecht, *Rudolph Virchow: Doctor, Statesman, Anthropologist*, University of Wisconsin Press, 1953.

W. Bulloch, *The History of Bacteriology*, Oxford University Press, 1938.

F. Grande, and M. B. Visscher, (eds.), *Claude Bernard and Experimental Medicine* [symposium, Minneapolis, 1965], Schenkman, 1967.

H. A. Kelly, *Walter Reed and Yellow Fever*, McClure, Phillips and Co., 1906.

H. A. Lechevalier, and M. Solotorovsky, *Three Centuries of Microbiology*, McGraw-Hill, 1965.

Nobel Lectures Including Presentation Speeches and Laureates' Biographies: Physiology or Medicine, 1922–1941, Elsevier, 1965, pp. 43–84.

G. M. D. Olmstead, and E. H. Olmstead, *Claude Bernard and the Experimental Method in Medicine*, Henry Schuman, 1952.

F. N. L. Poynter, (ed.), *Medicine and Science in the 1860s*, Wellcome Institute, 1968.

R. Virtanen, *Claude Bernard and His Place in the History of Ideas*, University of Nebraska Press.

Acknowledgements

Permission to reproduce the Readings in this volume is acknowledged from the following sources:

1 Blackwell Scientific Publications Ltd
2 Blackwell Scientific Publications Ltd
3 Harvard University Press and William Heinemann Ltd
4 The Regents of the University of California
5 The Johns Hopkins Press
6 Blackwell Scientific Publications Ltd
8 BPC Publishing Ltd
11 Edinburgh University Press
18 Stanford University Press
19 Stanford University Press
20 Dover Publications, Inc.
23 The C.V. Mosby Company
24 American Medical Association and Norman Simon

Index

History of Science Readings

Published simultaneously with this volume:

The Science of Matter

Edited by M. P. Crosland

The question 'What is matter?' is one of the most fundamental in science and has exercised the minds of the most eminent philosophers and scientists. Dr Crosland has provided a wide and general survey which spans several centuries: his collection of Readings presents a cross-section of the history of science, starting with the speculations of the Greeks and finishing with a paper on the conservation of parity. Many of the great figures in the history of science – Aristotle, Newton, Lavoisier, Faraday, Rutherford – are represented, and the Readings extend to the present-day world of elementary particles and anti-matter.

Augustine to Galileo

**Volume 1 Science in the Middle Ages
5th–13th Century**
**Volume 2 Science in the Later Middle Ages and
Early Modern Times 13th–17th Century**
A. C. Crombie

Augustine to Galileo is a two-volume survey of Western science in the
Middle Ages. Using recent research into original sources, Dr Crombie
traces the story of scientific theory and invention from its decay after
the collapse of the Roman Empire in the West to its full flowering in the
seventeenth century. He is primarily concerned with the internal
development of scientific thought and its practical achievements in
technology; but he also covers the more general influence of science on
the medieval world picture, in art, philosophy and theology. By
defining the questions they were intended to answer he makes even the
strangest of medieval scientific ideas readily intelligible; and he gives
much of the material necessary for analysing the development of
modern scientific thought.

The first volume describes the ideas about the natural world which were
current from the fifth to the twelfth centuries, and discusses the system
of scientific thought which was evolved from Greek and Arabic sources
in the thirteenth century. It also examines the relation of technical
activity to science throughout the Middle Ages.

The second volume describes the growth of medieval ideas on scientific
method, examines the increasing criticisms of the thirteenth-century
scientific system, and ends with a thorough analysis of the origins and
nature of the seventeenth-century Scientific Revolution.